Patterns of Life Force

Patterns of Life Force

A Review of the life and work of Dr Edward Bach
and his discovery of the Bach Flower Remedies

Julian Barnard

Bach Educational Programme

1987

By the same author

*

A Guide to the Bach Flower Remedies
[C.W. Daniel Company]

This is a useful introduction to the workings of
the Bach Flower Remedies

First published in Great Britain 1987
by Bach Educational Programme
© Julian Barnard 1987

ISBN 0 9506610 1 5

Set in 11 point Bembo
by Quorum Technical Services, Cheltenham
Printed and bound by Ebenezer Baylis   Worcester

Bach Educational Programme
P O Box 65
Hereford HR2 0UW

Contents

Dedication

This is given in thanks to the well of healing where all may come and draw freely of the love of life.

Thanks

My wife Martine has contributed substantially to this book. We have discussed the ideas of it together, she has helped provide much of the material and in every way has given of her generous love to it. Her sensitive advice has been combined with her warm encouragement. Without her it would not have been.

To others who have helped I equally give a heart-felt thank you: to Michele Sargoni for her research and assistance on many occasions; to Joy Southgate for her commitment and thoughtful encouragement; to Glenn Storhaug who helped with design and who gave freely of his most valuable advice; to my parents for their perennial willingness to help and for their loving kindness; to K. who has silently taught. And a special thank you to Nickie Murray who was my first contact with Bach's work and who has remained a true guide and to her husband Malcolm; both have given help and friendship.

Author's Preface

This is now complete. No, not perfect, not by a long way, but complete, dear reader, because you are now engaged with the process. Certain ideas are conveyed in this writing but their action is only useful in that they stimulate a response and review in you. There is not much here that can be taken on board and trotted out as learning but there is the possibility for a new perception, a different view of life. As such this is like water drawn from a well and you, if you will, may use it for whatever it seems good for.

In ancient times the well formed the centre of a settlement with families grouped around it. It was in the interests of all that it be free and kept in good order. The water was given by life, percolating through the earth and no one man could claim to own it. So it is with us. Edward Bach spoke of the flower remedies as "this God-sent Gift" and which of us would disagree? The nature of the gift is still becoming apparent as fifty years on we continue to draw benefit from his life work. The discoveries that Edward Bach made, however, are not, of themselves, the well. More of an apparatus, perhaps, a way of getting to the water.

It is my belief that we have only just begun to see the implications of Bach's work. The prospect is for a far greater development of human sensitivity and consciousness, a realisation of deeper potential in humanity. By this I do not mean that the clarity and simplicity of its use should be confused and muddled by extensions, rebuilding or redesigning the well – that would only muddy the water. Rather that we have the opportunity for a more profound understanding of what life is, by sharing the water.

The Bach Flower Remedies are used by many people in many different ways. They are taken as a simple healing medicine, used in conjunction with many different forms of treatment and different kinds of therapy. They have a following among many different people. But the flower remedies themselves are a way, stepping stones to understanding life. The more we understand Bach's ideas and come to terms with their implications the more we will see the true vision of what life might be when we can let go of our limitations. The glory of life is ever present but we may fail to perceive it.

So it can be said and recognised that whatever is true and resounding in this is not mine but drawn from life and whatever is limited and unfounded is only the result of my limitation.

Julian Barnard
October 1986
Herefordshire

1 · *Introduction*

The following is a quotation from Dr Edward Bach taken from his book *Free Thyself* written in 1932.

It is as simple as this, the Story of Life.

A small child has decided to paint the picture of a house in time for her mother's birthday. In her little mind the house is already painted; she knows what it is to be like down to the very smallest detail, there remains only to put it on paper.

Out comes the paint-box, the brush and the paint-rag, and full of enthusiasm and happiness she sets to work. Her whole attention and interest is centred on what she is doing – nothing can distract her from the work in hand.

The picture is finished in time for the birthday. To the very best of her ability she has put her idea of a house into form. It is a work of art because it is all her very own, every stroke done out of love for her mother, every window, every door painted in with the conviction that it is meant to be there. Even if it looks like a haystack, it is the most perfect house that has ever been painted; it is a success because the little artist has put her whole heart and soul, her whole being into the doing of it.

This is health, this is success and happiness and true service. Serving through love in perfect freedom in our own way.

So we come down into this world, knowing what picture we have to paint, having already mapped out our path through life, and all that remains for us to do is to put it into material form. We pass along full of joy and interest, concentrating all our attention upon the perfecting of that picture, and to the very best of our ability translating our own thoughts and aims into the physical life of whatever environment we have chosen.

Then, if we follow from start to finish our very own ideals, our very own desires with all the strength we possess, there is no failure, our life has been a tremendous success, a healthy and a happy one.

The same little story of the child-painter will illustrate how, if we allow them, the difficulties of life may interfere with this success and happiness and health, and deter us from our purpose.

The child is busily and happily painting when someone comes along and says, "Why not put a window here, and a door there; and of course the garden path should go this way." The result in the child will be complete loss of interest in the work; she may go on, but is now only putting somone else's ideas on paper: she may become cross, irritated, unhappy, afraid to refuse these suggestions; begin to hate the picture and perhaps tear it up: in fact, according to the type of child so will be the re-action.

The final picture may be a recognisable house, but it is an imperfect one and a failure because it is the interpretation of another's thoughts, not the child's. It is of no use as a birthday present because it may not be done in time, and the mother may have to wait another whole year for her gift.

This is disease, the re-action to interference. This is temporary failure and unhappiness: and this occurs when we allow others to interfere with our purpose in life, and implant in our minds doubt, or fear, or indifference.

The picture of a house is an expression of our being: our sense of ourselves. The way that we paint it is the way that we express the pattern of our life force.

Bach saw how the thoughts that we have for our life create its pattern. In this he made a link between our life and health and the way that we think and feel. Negative thoughts and interference, whether from ourselves or other people, create a distortion of the true pattern of what we aspire to be in life. He showed us that the thoughts that we have are powerful for the destruction, the maintenance and the creation of life.

2 · *The Birth → Death Process*

More than 200 thousand people are born each day. The circumstances vary from the very primitive to high-tech. While some of us were met first by the sight of the night sky others were amazed by the bright light of the operating theatre. No matter. We are all part of one humanity, born at this moment in this place and in no other. And for each of us the origins from which we take our form relate back to the same process: conception.

It is the miracle of life that everything is based upon this same process. We jokingly refer to the birds and the bees but that is just it! Behind all creation, existence, behind all living matter seen and unseen is the same process of life; we see its form in the time between birth and death; its substance is the material of life – life force. Life force, like a magnet, draws matter to itself. After conception the fertilised ovum divides and the single cells multiply to form the embryo. The life force that will become a human, a fish, a giraffe draws in the material to clothe itself for living in accordance with the pattern of its type of being. If the life force is strong then the body will be strong. If the life force is weak then the vehicle created for that life will be weak. If the life force dwindles and ceases then the form will be left, an uninhabited shell which will dissolve back into undifferentiated matter. Life declines into Death.

At any point during our conscious existence we may gauge the level of activity of life force in ourselves or in another. When the life force is strong in a plant it is visibly healthy, growing and prolific. If it is mature within its cycle of growth then the life force is gradually condensed into the seed or root in preparation for a new spring. If it is declining then the leaves fall, stems collapse and the plant will die. The process is the same throughout nature. We can observe the strength of the life force at the vegetable, animal or human levels.

How the life force works within us as human individuals is determined by many complex factors. While so called genetics may account for many of the physical characteristics of our children it is clear that other influences bear strongly upon the individual. Even when we share the same parents as children we are conceived in a different situation, a different time. What happens at conception and how the forces of life shape us may be difficult to assess. Being beyond the realms of physical measurement they are beyond the realms of conventional science, they belong to the metaphysical, the intangible. Yet every mother knows the circumstances of pregnancy and many can be sure of the moment of conception and the events that led to it. The more we are in tune with our body the more we hear its rhythms and messages of change. And without the need for astrology or mystery we can agree that the emotional circumstances that attend pregnancy and the creating of a new life form are instrumental in shaping it. Indeed it is the purpose of this book to illustrate how the strength of the life force is related to the emotional state of each and every one of us.

Broadly speaking the proposition is this. At the outset we are all pretty well strong in life force. But as the difficulties and experience of life on earth are encountered we are apt to close off from life and move towards death. Negative emotional states (fear, anger, indecision etc.) constrict the flow of vitality just as fatty deposits in the arteries constrict the flow of blood.

Life is about change and the facility for change. The greater the potential to continue living with the greatest potential for change, the greater the abundance of life. At the extreme we can see that extinction in life is the failure to adapt. If an organism cannot adapt to a change in climate it dies. The greater the potential for existence in a wide range of conditions the more prolific the life. Man is said to be an adaptable species in physical terms. But what holds true for the life potential physically is also applicable in other realms. We are more than a physical being and life is more than physical adaptability.

As a simple expression of this we all know how the child has a potential to become many things. "When I grow up", says the little boy, "I am going to be a racing driver, or an explorer...." The potential for either is there. But come 40 the potential for racing circuits seems to have faded and a wish to explore has a settled dust over it like schoolboy annuals left piled up in the attic. Either possibility could be reawakened however just as the potential for life can be rejuvenated. "Great-grandmother goes ballooning" brings a smile but it is always possible. Then again the potential for being an explorer can be developed in another way: as an explorer not of the outer world but of the inner regions of being – the landscape of our heart and mind. But such an exploration would need adaptability and the facility for change, it would require a greater potential for life. Thus old folk can be full of life, interested in new possibilities and discoveries and the young may close off in boredom. Life generally gives up on those who give up on it.

If life is the potential for change then a good illustration of it is a colony of bees. There may be 50 thousand insects in a hive. Each acts as a part of the whole, relating all its actions to the welfare and needs of the colony, fetching now nectar, now water, collecting pollen to feed the young or cleaning the cells in the wax brood combs for new eggs and larvae. The worker bees are not, as is often thought, obedient servants of the queen, rather they are individuals responding to the call of life. Because of this bees show an amazing ability to work with change always getting on with things as they are, responding directly to the present situation in accordance with the law of their being. If circumstances alter within the hive – maybe the queen dies or the hive is knocked over, maybe the day is very hot/cold or there is found to be insufficient space to store the incoming nectar – whatever happens the bees will work to continue the life of the colony in the most advantageous way. The pathway of life force between action and response is kept clear of difficulties. Of course there are occasions when bees cannot make up their minds but they are exceptional.

In terms of what bees do we can say they have a remarkable ability to adapt to change and life. But to perceive the life force at work in a hive it may be necessary to experience it, not as a set of theoretical probabilities (what will the bees do if this were to happen?) but as a living thing. Most people are afraid of bees because they might sting (life can be painful) but to sense the strength and beauty of this form of life we need to get close to it. We will feel it if we stop thinking of ourselves and we will rejoice in its strength if we stop feeling our strength threatened.

It is the same generally in life for us. If we are always thinking of ourselves we cannot experience the beauty of another being. If we see the other being as a threat to our strength and we react with a defensive posture to life, closing ourselves off in order to protect what we have, then we shall suffer. First we suffer because we miss the joy of relationship and communion with life and then we suffer because we close and constrict the movement of the life force within. It becomes suffocating, like breathing the stale air in a closed room. We suffer from ourselves as Dr Bach observed. Experience shows that the opposite reaction is the more rewarding. If we open ourselves to the experience of life we find happiness, strength and love. This is made more real in the difference between working with our head and working with our hearts. The opening of our hearts opens us to the experience of loving life.

A love of life is essential. When we suffer we think: how can I love life? But when we love life we will not be in suffering. It is a little bit the chicken and the egg. Which came first the suffering or the resentment? The suffering feeds the negative emotion (which constricts the life force) and the negative emotion causes the suffering. Which came first is academic.

When we act with a love of life we will only be concerned with the present way out of the problem: that is an instantaneous decision. And from that moment onwards, when we decide to love life, the potential and the future will change.

All nature works for the future. Bees collect their honey, trees and plants produce their millions of seeds, birds lay their eggs. Beneath the ground roots extend their shoots, nests of worms are knotted in obscurity while the moles tunnel blindly towards each other. It is through abundance that nature survives. This theme of generosity is familiar enough to us. But again it points to the way of life. Both on and in the land, the rivers and seas and in the air the myriad forms of creation show the process of life. We are a part of it.

At 1256 hrs today a child is being born. Now at this moment, as this child is writing. All the life stands before it in potential. In a room, in a town, in this part of a country is the physical location. In what other circumstances we can only guess. At the exact point from which we progress the easiest things to describe are the physical locations. The subtle world, the metaphysical, is not so clearly mapped out. The pattern of the life force, the way that life expresses itself for that being, is more ambiguous. We tend therefore to look at the physical components of life. So we can imagine the mother and the child within her; she working to bring to birth another being. How the child is born continues the story of its previous months of life. Is the birth traumatic? Is the mother anaesthetised? Is the father helping? Is the child unwilling? Are the others sympathetic, kind, loving or are they worried by their own difficulties and self-absorbed? Is the child born amid fears and uncertainty or surrounded by harmony and love? All these impressions will focus in the life of that small body.

The child is born. What happens next? Is it a disappointment (Oh dear, not another boy!)? Was it all a shock, not what we had expected? Our first reactions imprint themselves strongly and will probably continue to do so. If it is taken away from the mother how will they both react emotionally? Every event will be recorded as part of this child's life, whether it is remembered consciously or not. If we try to imagine the countless impressions that are registered by each of us, just in the first few weeks of life, we may wonder what could possibly hold such a record. The answer is that *we are* that record.

How the unique record of our lives play upon us we each know. Most of us, at some time in our life, try to discover the circumstances of our birth, just as a traveller will return to his native town. Equally we might recall the vivid moments of drama, the times of pain and sorrow, happiness and joy like streets and buildings in that town. We often walk in the lanes of our memories. Some of us have had the experience of working to revisit such places through the various techniques employed in workshops and groups. The journey of self-development often begins with a knowing of our past. But we should not spend too much time in the past. It is true that we have been through many experiences but they do not have to control us now. We are still alive and the story is not over yet. Life is for change and we can change our life now. The past may be the story of how we got here but it need not dictate what happens next.

3 · *Learning from Life*

We are in a time of great change. Seen in the context of a life time
our present age is filled with upheaval in every way, so much so
that we have all but become inured to it – social, religious,
political, economic, educational and moral change are so
commonplace that we are getting quite used to the idea. We are
coming to expect and even to crave novelty. In science we wait
restlessly for new marvels of daring and delicacy whether in
space flight, in biotechnology or atomic physics. In the
marketplace new products succeed each other so that after 2 or 3
years a machine design is said to be obsolete. Not to be new is to
be nothing. What are we to do?

In human terms this thrust for change causes us considerable difficulties. In times of great stability we form attachments
emotionally to certain idea structures. They help to hold and
mediate the life force like a vessel, giving stability and constancy to our activity. But in times of change these idea
structures act against us because of the attachment that we have
to them. We find it difficult to look with a free objectivity at
what is happening because we are held in the shell of past
patterns. In some cases this shell has become so thick and
unresponsive that the life force within it is unable to move
outwardly at all. Nothing can come in, no relationship with
external forces is possible. The life becomes like a stubborn and
unrelenting opponent of change. Bigotry is everywhere.

Such patterns lock us in positions of difficulty. They are
carried by individuals, in families and within communities and
nations. They are the idea structures that determine barriers,
blocks, gulfs, impossibilities. We all hold them in varying

degrees and in different forms according to our natures. And we hold to them passionately feeding their structure and stricture with our emotional responses like a mollusc secreting the substance of the shell in which it lives. We can see the activity of these emotional patterns by asking ourselves a few simple questions. The questions could relate to religion, politics, sex, education, family obligations, sexual roles, childhood and so on.

Within family units these patterns of behaviour appear to stream in from the past through the generations of the family. Like the obligations of revenge the emotions are often set by inheritance. The ideas that structure the assumptions of power or the aspiration to improvement or the acceptance of poverty are bred into us. As such they become imbued with an emotional charge for us in our family unit where they may be completely absent for our neighbour.

In a wider context we can watch these emotional patterns at work in the many religious and sectarian wars that are being fought at the present time or the countless theatres of ideological struggle throughout the world. We see people who will seek to destroy life for the sake of maintaining or strengthening an idea. Nor should we imagine that we ourselves are mere spectators in this situation. Let us gauge our own responses to local conflicts and our own struggles as well. In it all we can observe the same thing: life is not considered as important as these idea-shells that rule our emotions and our actions. Life is cheap when it is so little in evidence. We see our opponents not as life forms but as animated masks, often more mechanical than human. Or else we don a mask ourselves to disguise our humanity and commit atrocity.

The experience of meeting, not a human being but a set of programmed or patterned responses is both the product and the reason for our contemporary reductionist view of life (when we see ourselves not as the greatest we might be but as the smallest that can be proved achievable by all). To some, man is a machine, but a machine for what? It is a disturbing line of thought for many of us. But when we meet another person who will not meet our eyes, who will not look us straight, we are encountering not a free life-spirit but a pattern of emotional fixity and we should be warned.

In times of change these patterns, karmic shells as they are called, will be assaulted. Sometimes, if they are no longer supplied with life force they will become brittle and fall away. Times of personal change may lead to such an opening to life. Sometimes a little conflict will jolt the shell and release us. For others a jolt is not enough and many blows are needed to crack open the shell. For each of us the story is similar and yet unique.

The shells are fed by a variety of emotional patterns although the process is similar. We are bound by such things as fear, pride, greed, jealousy or hatred; by negative emotions that are based upon past life experience. These shells prevent us from meeting new life experiences freely (we are prejudiced – we prejudge them). When the shells are broken we have to face life without the protection of this casing as a delicate kernel of life force ready to grow. It is a high risk business.

Because of the dangers of being so apparently vulnerable we generally scamper into the shelter of our shells. When we face what appear to be threatening questions about our life or existence we take refuge in available belief and accepted philosophy. Of course, this may be the genuine product of our life experience. Yet if it is we will find it no shell nor shelter but a radiating centre of love for life. More often though the refugee will find it is a way of giving authority to other people who will hold sway through the power of their certainty.

The man who holds the sway in ideas holds more power than the military chieftain because he holds the key to people's hearts or rather the emotional patterns and karmic shells. Religion, in times of change, leads to disagreement and alienation. In an age of stability the problem does not arise because the external world conforms consistently with the internal idea. But when changes occur our inflexibility makes for dogmatism and blind belief. One man's religion is another man's prejudice. We rush to join the One True Way Club whose members are certain they alone know the Real Truth. The more difficult a thing is to prove, the more we feel the need to be right and the more threatened we are by alternative points of view. Ideas can become very destructive forces.

For some the answer lies in happy ignorance: I would rather be a goldfish, mouthing water in a bowl. But that is just another kind of shell, the shell of ignorance, a way of avoiding life. And for the real fish there is no such reality as it encounters life force and life experience at its own level of being. For us there is really no other choice. We can only learn to work with life or come to terms with the consequences of refusal. The consequences of refusal are death.

We stand in this balance between life and death. It is the nature of our existence. For each of us the condition of our being reflects the balance of these forces. And for each the story of our life has led to our being here now. To know why we are in this present situation we must make true observation of what has gone before. If we see it for what it is we may be able to understand how we got here and how the forces of life have arranged themselves in our body. To move forward from that position, to observe and learn the lessons that are there in the past experience and to apply them to the present is to understand why. But for that 'why' to have reality it must be free of prejudice, dogma and preconceived ideas. It must be free from the influence of karmic patterns.

Without a structure of ideas though we are apparently unprotected, vulnerable. We are then thrown back upon the resources of the heart. Our love of life alone can sustain us. Like a refugee we are dependent upon human kindness and the generosity of life. But unencumbered we may yet be the ones who survive.

4 · *The Riddle of Nature* [1]

When we look at architecture it is surprising to see how varied the forms of building are. While in the western world we prefer hard shells of concrete and stone others make light-weight structures of canvas and bamboo. The massive edifices of our modern cities (twentieth century cathedrals) are supposed to be a mark of civilisation and enlightened thought. A comparison of building technology and idea structures would be rewarding. The Bedouin in his tent allows the outside breeze to circulate, like the Red Indian he is closer to the land. In Japan the bamboo and paper walls are designed for flexibility. The buildings that a culture erects are monuments to their thought and speak of their relationship to life. A bank vault is as deadly as the grave. We live therefore more or less in harmony with nature and we build in a way that displays our need to dominate the natural world or our willingness to accept it.

It is said that if you wish to find out what you are like you should look around you. Look at where and how you live. Look at what is considered of value and important. We are like what we are. It is thought that we are what we eat; equally we are what we think and we become what we do. The nature of our activity will shape our being.

Sometimes it may be possible to live and forget that the world exists outside. The vision of Metropolis is one where man and machine are the totality of life. But it is foolish to think that we can survive for long without the natural world from which we obtain all life sustenance. The contemplative thinker in his cell (an area of life force surrounded by a barrier) and the business tycoon in his office may have this in common that they both withdraw so far into their thoughts that ideas dominate their perception of life and they become blind. Our attachment to what money or any other idea can bring is just another shell – as has been suggested it is these emotional attachments that need to be cleared if we are to perceive the truth.

Because our lives are dominated by our emotional attachment to ideas we are blind to the consequences of our actions. This blindness becomes habitual and we no longer see what we are doing. We have lost the ability to discriminate between what is helpful and what is damaging to life. We think that we are rather separate from life and can therefore prey upon it but because we are part of life we cannot act independently (so long as we are alive!). The idea of nuclear arsenals that can destroy the world not just once but ten times over is absurd. Absurd in just the same way that a man should have ten times more food than he can eat. It is not a moral offence so much as it is indiscriminate, like deafness (ab- + surdus, deaf or dull; O.E.D.). Without ears and eyes our balance is gone: we swing between choices unable to decide, lacking the centre from which to act.

So there is the need to return to a simplicity where those ideas we hold to, like a tent, can provide shelter and yet be carried as we travel; ideas that allow for life and so for change. Something with tensile strength and flexibility which will not crystallize and harden into a shell and constrict us. The idea of life force is like this. Not so much an edifice as a plank across the canyon.

Anthropologists who study the life and beliefs of different cultures can observe how many societies live in such a way that their lives and practices are not in conflict with the natural world. Rituals that we might call primitive serve to remind such people of the relationship they have with nature. Their thoughts about life and the forms that follow upon those thoughts are not set in conflict with the world in which they live; their actions apparently have a simple fitness in them, they are appropriate. As change overtakes these societies they flounder in confusion. Western thinking as much as western materialism breaches the integrity of the culture.

It is not so far different for us. By instinct we are pantheistic seeing God in all things, just as God is in life. As children we are drawn by simple joy to experience and love life. If left without interference how might things develop? But the experienced are jealous of innocence and will not allow it. So we begin to localise experience (according to karmic patterning again) and come to see some things as holy and others as profane. For both we build temples and so enshrine the polarity. And these temples are no light-weight affairs.

All this is because our life and what we do is a literal reflection of what we are. What we build and what we cherish is a reflection of our inner state of mind. Indeed external life is one and the same as internal life. It is only because we are sold on the idea of conflict, polarity, duality that we would ever see it otherwise. But life is one, not two!

To see this however we must think with the heart and look with a fresh eye upon our existence. It is not so easy for the conditioning is strong. Look out of the window and you will see what you are – for the world reflects to us our nature.

Two men look out through prison bars
The one sees mud, the other stars.

We choose what we see and select from the external world what will reinforce the world picture that we have formed internally. This world picture is decided by our emotional attachment to ideas. Beauty, after all, is in the eye of the beholder. The critical eye will see only ugliness and find fault, the disapponted only disappointment.

In the world of nature there is a riddle. That world is made of the same material as we are and it carries in it the imprint of the same force of patterning, consequently we are like it. The riddle? Phrase it how you will but basically it is this: the world and our idea of life are one and the same...the world is just the expression of an idea.

Everything that exists must be conceived. What is conceived in a physical state must first be conceived in the mind, in the imagination. This conception is a thought form. It is the form that can be filled by life force to bring a living substance into existence. Thought forms are held by all life structures that have or hold life force. We are, ourselves, a thought form, just as we are conceived. The world as we see it, that too is a thought form. Plants, trees, grass, flowers, these are all thought forms of the planet. Seeds are a condensing of one individual thought form that has the potential through the activation of life force to grow into a full expression of that idea. From a grain of mustard may grow a great plant.

That we recognise such a state of affairs as self-evident should not surprise us. It is a statement of the obvious. But humans seem to have forgotten just what human beings are and what their relationship is with the natural world. The memory, however, is near at hand in all our language and imagery. We have just been using it. This after all is the seed of an idea. It may grow in the fertile soil of the individual reader into a strong plant, bearing fruit.

In literature nature is always analogous to human experience. Writers have unerringly recognised that the human estate is reflected in and a reflection of the images of the natural world. Ideas take root in the mind, a reflective mood is like still water, sweet thoughts are flowers, others rank weeds. Troubles cloud the mind, children have a sunny disposition, some activities are fruitful others nipped in the bud; we weather storms, have hopes dampened, cultivate good habits or have thoughts scattered to the winds; passions burn and ardour is fanned; old age is autumnal, youth like spring; we are thrifty like squirrels, collectors with a magpie instinct, chatter like sparrows, proud as peacocks, frightened as a mouse or greedy as pigs; we are shy violets, rosy cheeked or fresh as a daisy.

But more than this the natural world bears within an exact counterpart to our own life experience. Nature constantly provides the illustration by which we recognise a picture of the truth; it is in nature that our questions can be answered. As Job said:

Speak to the earth and it shall teach you.[2]

The world is the only example that we have – there is no other. Where else is there that we may learn, what other expression of thought can we have? Without our seeing of the world (or our report of it) what language do we have for thought? Since thought is so far a part of us how can we but conclude that the world, planet, earth and all that is therein is a part of us too. Actually whether we are part of it or it is part of us is hardly the point: we are one with life.

Contemporary thinking will not work well with this concept. We have grown used to the idea that man and nature are separate entities. We see life in terms of stratification, hierarchies and evolutionary levels. Needless to say man is on the top in each case. Like adolescents we imagine we have outgrown our parents and that we are now quite able to manage this life estate. But the farmer does not create the seed, nor the plant geneticists, they are merely tampering with life. The great processes of life were there long before we discovered genetic engineering and will continue long after all human empires are laid waste. Whether we (humanity) continue with life depends pretty much upon what we do now.

In many respects the thought forms of the planet and the thought forms of mankind are compatible. The difficulty arises when our thought forms become destructive and start to exclude the thought forms of the planet. The result causes planetary damage. At a simple practical level the thought form that creates toxic waste is destructive to life. People know this and will not willingly encounter radiation. But while pollution, drugs, chemicals and so on poison life they are minor damage compared to the effect of actual thought forms themselves. Negative thought forms as we might call them, thoughts that act against life, are the real danger to the planet and to life. We can witness their effects in several ways: again look out of the window and we can see what man's thought forms have created; then let us look at ourselves and recognise how the thought forms that create us are reflected in us and thirdly, though it is more difficult, we can perceive how the negative thought forms of humanity dislocate the thought forms of the planet.

This last matter shows first as the withdrawal of a planetary thought form. If a particular plant or animal species becomes extinct the thought form that created it is no longer supplying the vessel for that life. Equally though, there are certain species that become more prolific in response but these species are the predators and the dominant, often damaging forms that are hostile to the ecological balance. It is more than a matter of conservation, however. When people steal the eggs of rare breeding birds it creates publicity but as far as the thought form goes it is already too late. Life cannot survive as a zoo species.

In fact the natural species on this planet are being withdrawn from life at a fantastic rate. But still the world looks pretty much the same as it was and we might imagine that all was well. But the time scale for the planet is vast and we have yet to understand it. If the planet actually changed its mind (thought forms) it would take a long time for us to realise it and we can only speculate as to whether those thought forms would be compatible with the thought for human life. The result undoubtedly would be a great change for humanity.

At present we need only look at the earth to see a reflection of our state. Just as the poet sees the light of reason and the dawn of hope within the imagery of nature so we can see the torture and degradation of the natural world as a statement of our situation. We need to realise that toxic thoughts are toxic waste, that rapacious greed despoils the land, that emotional desolation creates a wasteland, that war and destruction are born in the fear of our hearts and in the cruelty of our thoughts.

So too we can recognise that hope springs eternal, that where the gentle rain of reason falls the hard earth will soften. Where the sunshine of joy and love can warm us the seeds of new life will germinate and if we allow them to grow the herbs of the field can flower for our healing and for health.

5 · *Drawing Breath*

The most important, or at least the most essential, processes in life are automatic. They occur without conscious thought, by virtue of life's natural activity: like breathing. If we had actually to learn consciously the chemical processes of digestion before we could utilise food we might not survive for long. If we had always to remember to breathe there might be time for little else. If the mind was totally occupied by the thought of taking breath, holding it, exchanging the gases and other life-giving substances and then expelling the air what would happen to argument, anxiety, self-pity or fear? What fills the mind tends to fill the life. Indeed it is the basis of some meditative practices that if we quiet the mind and stop the chit-chat of thoughts by concentrating upon a single thing then we will experience a greater tranquillity in our life. The heart does not suffer from the same restlessness as the mind. That is why, when we think with our hearts we find simplicity and clarity.

People who study animal behaviour observe the intricacy of the instinctive patterning that animals use. These behaviour patterns are apparently innate to individual species – herring gull chicks peck at a red spot like that on the parents' beak expecting food, spiders spin webs through a natural design skill rather than through experimentation. Human behaviourists observe similar patterns in our ways of living. This does not demean the status of human or bird but it invites the observation that instinctive behaviour plays an important part in all life forms. If everything in life was always experimental the result would be chaos. Instinct, as we call it, mediates between innovation and closely ordered behaviour. In human terms there has been a tendency to see instinct as crude and evidence of low intelligence. Instinctive behaviour in animals conversely is seen as evidence of a higher animal intelligence. Neither view is accurate because of a false view of intelligence.

Life learns a pattern through repetition. Repetition leads to ordered behaviour – I do this because it is what I always do! Instinct comes into play when ordered behaviour is made part of the life pattern for that species. It is part of the thought form that creates the spider or the gull. As such it is inbuilt, innate, they are born with it. For humans the same is true. We do not learn to breathe, it is instinctive, just as sucking is or crawling.

Other behaviour patterns can become almost instinctive within a family unit if the activities are repeated through generations. A baby follows the demonstrated behaviour of parents. At 18 months a whole vocabulary of gesture and sound exactly mimics the adults. The toddler will stand, look and move just like the parents. Thus we carry 'sign stimuli' as surely as the herring gull. This gesture means food, this tone of voice means bed. We do with our children what our parents did with us (as evidenced by child abuse). Not always: it is possible to take a conscious decision to change but generally this is the process.

These instinctive behaviour patterns are very strong and we are strongly attached to them. Once formed they are difficult to break. If it is said that you cannot teach an old dog new tricks it is because the patterns are most strongly learned in early life. Yet another phenomenon of animal behaviour is of interest here. It is called enemy learning. A group of birds will call in alarm at the sight of a predator. When a hawk appears (or even the shadow of one) the mother hen will call in her chicks. A cry of alarm will go through the local bird populace, the threat is general. But it is not necessary for every individual to see the hawk, the sound of the alarm call alone will alert them. In laboratory experiments groups of birds have been taught that harmless objects are predators by associating the object with the alarm call. This kind of enemy learning is a strong force within human communities as well as in family behaviour patterns.

How does it work? Suppose the family meet a situation that the parents view as a threat, suppose the door bell rings. Well, what kind of a threat is that? It is unexpected, Mum jumps, Dad thinks "I hope it isn't...", fear, anxiety, apprehension all round. The children learn the pattern: always fear the worst, a knock at the door is ominous. When the door is opened, however, it turns out to be a welcome visitor, one bearing gifts even. The children now study the adult response: suddenly the anxious glances have been exchanged for the nervous chatter of relief. The pattern is being imprinted.

The imprinting is far stronger however if it is attached to specific objects or ideas. The inexplicable fear or attraction for beards, blondes, tall or short people is often built in through this family patterning. It should be noted too that if a single experience is strong enough it needs no repetition to become indelibly imprinted – sexual abuse in particular is like this and fears and phobias that carry from the one experience are many.

Thus we learn from our family group a way of reacting to life. It will be superimposed upon and modify the other inherited patterns that we already carry with us. We will then learn a type of breathing in accord with what we see adults do. When enemy learning is being imprinted we will also learn a multitude of other responses. Some responses are basic instinctive like the urge to urinate, what is called a fight or flight response. Others are strictly local to the family group: when frightened we may eat or not eat, breathe fast and shallow or virtually stop breathing, shout, cry, sing, laugh, indeed the responses can be so varied as to be contradictory and difficult to recognise as a fear-related response.

All of these behaviour patterns engage our emotions and although the ideas that trigger them are instinctive rather than intellectual they bind themselves as part of the karmic pattern of our life and become fused into the karmic shell.

Another way in which these patterns build can be seen in personal relationships. If there is disagreement some resolve must be reached. Either we compromise, change our viewpoint or go into a win/lose position. If it becomes win/lose then it is a trial of strength; who can impose their will, who can get their own way? In such a conflict all kinds of ammunition can be used and the trial of strength will certainly activate many of the learned patterns from childhood. Eventually a victor will emerge. The conflict now is over apparently. But what of the vanquished, how will they deal with the situation? They respond with prejudice so that any comparable situation is prejudged to be unfavourable and attitudes are developed that will pervert any truthful meeting in the future. Prejudice in turn creates counter prejudice in the other so that pretty soon characterisation speaks to characterisation and all true meeting is prevented. These prejudices are inevitably passed on within family groups, role models are perpetuated with all their attendant limitations.

So the inheritors (the children) are assailed on a broad front. First they see a set of behaviour patterns upon which they model their bodies: these show a way of working intinctively in posture, breathing etc. Then they are given a set of idea prejudices which dispose them to view life in a particular way – all men do this...all women are that.... Thus bodies, emotions and ideas are given shape. Well, yes, of course they may be positive models, good ones, but then our prejudices will determine what is good. Which of us deliberately would give our children negative patterning? Which of us having a child who asked for bread would give him a stone? Alas, we can all too rarely tell the difference.

What then can change it? The clue lies in the breathing. For by observing the breath we can see the first movements of life and activity. When we can observe the natural pattern of our breathing then we can observe when it varies. The variation in breathing patterns at least can make us aware of our varying responses to what we encounter in life and we may be able to recognise what is happening within us. We need to become conscious of these instinctive responses. We already have some experience of this as part of our general vocabulary: when surprised we have 'a sharp intake of breath', we 'hold our breath' in anticipation and when tension passes we 'give a sigh of relief '. The process of respiration defines life in so far as it leads to an exchange of that which is outside with that inside. Without change there is no life. So the way we breathe is significant of the way that we encounter life.

Other body processes are equally essential, the action of the heart, for instance. The physical heart acts to circulate what is already internal. But when we look at the metaphysical action of the heart we can see it as the organ that mediates our emotional responses to the exchanges we have internally and externally. Where is the seat of love? Why, in the heart of course. And it is our love or lack of it that determines our emotional responses. An open heart meets life with joy; if we love life our responses are happy and positive, we breathe easy. But when we meet with a difficulty that triggers our instinctive responses, where the learned behaviour is brought into play (when we respond not with openness but with the fixity of karmic patterning) the heart is not open, rather it closes off. The sensation, for it has actually a feeling attached to it, is a framing of the heart, like a freeze-frame facility in a movie film. Then the heart constricts and the flow of life force is stopped. At the same time the breathing constricts and altogether the being stops free exchange with the environment around. Like a snail withdrawing into its shell so we retreat into stereotyped behaviour.

If we keep breathing and try hard to keep the heart open with a love and trust of life we may avoid these prejudiced responses. As for the karmic shells they can be broken by shock it is true but they can also be discharged if we simply do not feed them life. One such exercise leads to the thought "like what it doesn't like" where "it" is the characterisation of the karmic pattern. But if we simply do not continue our emotional attachment to the pattern we will starve it and in time it must surely grow brittle and fall away. This may be helped if the life situation is changed, for change induces new activity and a movement of life force. Our way of dealing with such a problem suggests the real nature of intelligence: it is not a fixed quantity to be calibrated, it is rather a qualitative ability to respond to life and the changes that it may bring. To the heart this may be instinct but to the mind an act of conscious intent.

6 · *Your Body Speaks its Mind*

"Well I couldn't stand it anymore ," I said, "I'm going to give
him a piece of my mind..." Ah! What kind of a gift will that be?
Usually something fairly unpleasant if the image runs true to
form. We do not always fill the mind with sweet thoughts.
Certainly that sentence evokes the picture of an outraged
person who has delivered a parcel of abuse to the neighbour.
We might quickly build an imaginary drama but somehow it is
already familiar enough. When tensions and conflict develop
we have many ways of dealing with them and sure not
everyone will take the path of action. But whether we keep our
negativity to ourselves or pass it on to others the common
experience is one of dissatisfaction with life.

Our thoughts reflect what we feel about life. If we love life
we have loving thoughts that are sweet and fragrant. If we
resent our situation and feel unfairly treated by life our thoughts
will be bitter and acrid. And what we share of our mind with
others will be in accord with what we carry in our thoughts. We
may convey the pure clear light of reason, the cold dispassion-
ate thoughts of the uncaring, the crystalline thoughts of the
unyielding which are beautiful but without life or the scattered
thoughts of the confused.

As thoughts come to speech we will see their quality. Noble
or beautiful thoughts are not reserved to fancy language but
they will make any language fine and beautiful. Similarly cruel
thoughts will corrupt the fairest words. The force of the
thought that is behind the words will show through and we
recognise this instinctively as hypocrisy. Some words create
destructive force patterns by their very sound and should be

avoided. Certain words that are frequently used in situations of stress for instance can both reflect and induce the difficulty. Sound has both a creative and destructive force and like thought it influences our bodies. And we may recognise here that just as thought can act to distort the pattern of the life force so too thought can act to realign the pattern of the life force.

We each form a picture of life which shows us to be more or less satisfied with how it is. Our thoughts are specific to our individual life story but the principles guiding them will be the same. We think about that which is either inside of ourselves or outside and it either makes us happy or unhappy. The unhappy person therefore may be unhappy because they do not like the way the external world exists ("I want that situation altered") or because their inner life makes them feel miserable ("I feel depressed"). Then again somebody may be happy with them-selves internally ("Yum, yum, I am eating a lovely cake") or externally ("What a beautiful day..."). These four states are equivalent to the four traditional temperaments: choleric, melancholic, phlegmatic and sanguine. We can act in accord-ance with any of them at differing times although we may have a disposition towards one more than another in our way of thinking.

The way that we fill our minds with thoughts is generally seen as a private affair. And in detail it is generally so. But the quality of thought will show itself and be read rather clearly in the body where although we keep our lips sealed the mind will speak: Your Body Speaks its Mind. A smile can be translated into many ideas but a real smile always shows a kind of pleasure and happiness. It may be a welcoming smile (thought:I am happy to see you) or a tight, satisfied smile (thought: there, I knew I would be right), an enigmatic smile (the Mona Lisa and who can guess her thought?) or a quiet secret smile of inner pleasure when we think of one we love. So too the mouth betrays our grief and sorrow, it may be twisted into a snarl of rage or contempt, it may pout or ponder: as our feelings and thoughts change so too the lips form and reform into an expressive pattern. In time the form of the habitual thought produces the form habitual to the mouth.

What is true for the mouth is true for the rest of the face. In the eyes we read boredom, indifference, suspicion, detachment or deference. They blaze with anger, sparkle with interest, gaze with longing, are dull with fear. As the mind in fear is unsteady and hovers in apprehension so the eyes wander and will not settle. In the nose or chin we can read the thoughts too: why else do the proud look down their noses and the willful stick out their chin. Again the body responds to what is in the mind. Children are expert at learning this body language and before the thought can form, the instinctive responses interpret the signs and learn the vocabulary of this form of speech, as we have already discussed.

Other parts of the body are as vocal in the declaration as the face. The stiffness of the neck and back display the thoughts of pride and self-esteem. The bombastic belly shows the urge to self-aggrandisement and power. A bowed back shows one bent by burdens, carrying guilt, grief, the cares of others or the load of responsibility. Hunched shoulders and a compressed chest speak of fears and lack of confidence. Those who suffer confusion in the mind display a confusion in the body and as the thoughts go without balance and direction like a chicken being chased so too the body shows arms and legs that lack the coordination of a clear purpose. As a body-builder has but the one thought of rippling muscle so we daily exercise and perform to create the outward expression of our life. A mind that is closed and patterned by obedience to a single thought shows as an automaton that marches like a drill soldier; a mind that is watchful and receptive demonstrates poise, balance and alertness ... actively calm and calmly active.

All of our life then speaks through our body and the way that we live. A man tortured in body or mind carries the scars. A fakir with his shrivelled arm held aloft demonstrates the result of fixed thought forms held perpetually in place. Each body speaks its life. The patterns of the past condition the way we act now – the karmic shells constrict and channel our life force into a moulded course of activity. Like a river that cuts and undercuts the bank as it meanders through the land so our life force flows within the channel of our behaviour. Where we meet soft shale or clay the river spreads and widens, where there is a band of hard rock it rebounds into a tight rush of turbulence. When the winter floods bring debris washing down from the upper reaches the river may burst its banks and reform its channel. The old water course may be left as stagnant pools; lakes and marshes may form behind a dam. If we examine the landscape we will see that it is in a state of change. It lives: it must change. That change displays structure, process and stage. The structure is the pattern of the idea form and its material; the process is the way that it now is being shaped, and the stage denotes the extent to which it has moved within the process. A river profile can be drawn that is like a life, the scenery like the thought forms that surround us, the rain and sun like the gifts of life. As the spring flows from the hillside, filled with water that fell upon the mountain so through all the villages and towns the river of life flows to come at last to unite with the sea.

7 · *It's not Where We Are – it's Where We Are At*

This year, 1986, is the centenary of the birth of Edward Bach. One hundred years ago on September 24th he was born at Moseley near Birmingham in the heart of England. He lived a convenient 50 years and died in the evening of November 27th 1936. Like many who lived and worked in the first decades of this century he saw the great upheaval of the western world and the revolutions of society. It is customary to notice change by reference to aeroplanes and motor cars and certainly during his life he saw the technological stirrings of the 20th century. As a young man before the Great War he must have seen the first flights and may have shared the general enthusiasm for innovation. He arrived in London just in time to see the last horse-drawn omnibus and during the next 20 years (he lived in London 1910-1930) he cannot but have noticed the effect of radio and telephone upon the city institutions. We now witness the electronic revolution and computerisation, it is another surge of change.

While Bach studied medicine and qualified as a medical doctor the great landmarks of modern science were being mapped. In the first discovery of radiation by Becquerel (a name we all have good reason to remember) when Bach was 10 years old, the workings of modern physics were implicit. And indeed some of the workings of modern medicine. The ideas of 50 years ago become the reality of today. And it is only to state the obvious to observe that the century since Bach was born has seen the discovery and development of devices that have radically changed the context of life for every one of us.

The changes in physical and social circumstances, however, are less significant than the changes in ideas themselves. We see the outward show of new design and can plot a sort of progress by the speed records and space flights but they are less significant for life than the changes in thought. Thought it is true can create those material forms but the greatest alteration has come in relation to how we think about ourselves. This has been born out of a slow change in the great thought forms that control the psyche of mankind. These dictate that in the cultures of different ages mankind has seen a differing reality: the world view of the Greek being different to that of the Roman, the medieval churchman seeing a different picture of the hierarchy of being to the philosophers of the 18th century. Whilst there is debate as to when we encountered the nadir in the great cycles of cosmic thought it is generally agreed that we are now on the upswing and we are moving progressively from the dark ages of materialism.

A signal of the changing consciousness of people in western society during the last hundred years is the coming of the term 'psychological'. In the 1880's a few philosophers hinted at the workings of the subtle mind. The Romantic Poets who wrote in terms of longing for the soul guessed at the workings of the psyche. But most people knew only the simple injunctions of religion. Few indeed saw anything beyond the stability of a society based upon material wealth and the personal power that derived from it. Today our outlook may still appear to be materialistic but our world view has been enlarged in great measure. Ideas only slowly become acceptable to the public consciousness. As we have come to understand the subtlety of electricity so our consciousness too has changed. If we were to walk now into the street and ask "what is psychology?" we can be sure that the vast majority would understand the question and give a reasonable answer.

This shift in perception has now become universal. Rather as the colonialists of the 19th century explored and occupied the physical world so in the 20th century we have explored and colonised the psychological world. The effects of this are apparent even in the comic books of our children: the moral stories of missionaries in Africa have given way to robot transformers in a world where not all is what it seems. The moral struggle of good and evil now takes place within the geography of our minds.

As we know the foundation stones of our modern understanding of the mind were laid in Austria and Switzerland by Freud and Jung. It is unfair to suggest that they were entirely original: Mesmer had worked in Austria too a hundred years before but now everyone knows these names and they are among the folk-heroes of modern thought. Yet whether history is made by individuals is debatable and the event that helped so many people into the recognition of the psyche was the First World War. Again it was the poets who were first into the field (Graves and Sassoon, for instance) but almost every household encountered the effect of shock, mental trauma and fatigue and saw the way their loved ones must deal with it. War was no longer the noble pursuit of young braves but a horrific initiation into torments of the mind. It was not a pointless slaughter, however: as the shells rained down upon the trenches the karmic shells of a generation were cracking open.

With the great changes that shook Western Europe in World War I came the opportunity to look afresh at life patterns. It is true that in some measure the karmic shells were carefully reasssembled and glued back together again so that the appearance of normality was resumed. But as we know from history the flood of change was washing at the steps of many of the grand monuments of authority. A simple recognition of humanity began to replace the blind assumptions of privilege.

For some the shock of the war left them incapable. A new medical term came to describe them as 'shell-shocked'. Nothing much could be done to help but observation concluded that when the mind was strained beyond all bearable limits the body responded in peculiar and unpredicatable ways. There was the dawn of an idea that our mental state affected our physical state. Like any idea it can be turned for good or ill and from such a seed could grow the horrors of brain washing and the basis for a new medicine.

Historians have suggested that a second world war was inevitable after the way that the first was ended. Between the wars two great forces seem to have been at work. The one was to file claims for justice and a proper resolution to grievances (social problems and national socialism) the other to persuade people to see humanity in a different way. During these years many great teachers worked in the west trying to change the consciousness (psychological outlook) of their followers. Gurdjieff, Steiner, Annie Besant and the Theosophists for instance. As grieving families tried to contact their dead loved ones spiritualism grew popular: accounts of life beyond the grave were provided by *A soldier* and other spirit guides.

These sort of influences changed the thinking of a generation; unseen in many ways but none the less potent for that. Perhaps the most significant teacher came to the west on the first passenger ship to leave India after the war. It docked in New York in late September 1920. Swami Yogananda brought a spiritual knowledge from the east that might transform the consciousness of mankind – the ancient creedless teachings of *Kriya Yoga*.

At about this time many texts of oriental philosophy and religion began to be available in new translation. First they were seen as being of scholarly interest but gradually they dissolved like honey into the warm water of our soul consciousness. They held a hope for the future, a possibility that new ways of thought from ancient thought might offer insight to the perplexity of western rationalism.

After the Second World War a generation were born to whom the journey to the east, whether in book or in body was a

strong attraction. If a list of names can serve to remind us it is
such as Jung, *I Ching*, Lao Tzu, Herman Hesse and Tolkien
who have shaped our thoughts. The 'love generation', hippies,
flower children *et al* are the offspring of the spiritual renewal
that took place in the years between the wars. Even the interest
in wholemeal food and a vegetarian diet started then. We have
been the inheritors of the aspirations and thought forms of the
grandfathers: ideas germinate for a generation before they
grow in force.

Instability in times of change produces diversity of thought:
we are not all sold on the notion of mysticism and for that we
may be thankful. But it is helpful to recognise that we work
within the context of certain thought forms. The products of
scientific modernism (call it what you will) are all too well
known to enumerate. So the ideas that stand as alternative in
our society seem the more interesting. Of course what value we
place upon them is a matter for the individual to decide.

The advent of psychology, a science of the mind, has
spawned a host of areas of study that relate to our physical and
mental states. As science was once the total study of all matter
and has now become a number of specialisations so too has the
study of the mind proliferated. An instinct of our time seems to
be this urge to divide things up into categories and parts so that
we become immersed in smaller and smaller details. By
becoming special (specialisation) we hope to find identity. But
another form of thought suggests that a whole being is greater
than its assembled parts and that we cannot hope to understand
life if we dissect it and cut it into pieces.

As ordinary human beings (not specialists) what are we to
make of this matter? It appears that no sooner is something
discovered than it becomes another department of study to
which we are not allowed access, the doors being locked by
jargon and scientific terminology. The findings of the specialist
are published as new knowledge which a generation later we
are expected somehow to understand as it is taught to our

children as scientific fact. The difficulty is that we have no general formula for life to which we can refer matters. In times gone by we might use religion but it is clear that science and religion have moved to worlds apart.

No sooner had we come to accept the idea of the psyche than we had to contend with differing opinion, competing schools of thought with differing theories, claims and counter claims. It is difficult for anybody who is not in the game (a specialist) to know what to make of it. In fact, of course, what we try to do is to get on with our lives and ignore it all. That is fine until something goes wrong. If our car breaks down we go to a mechanic (specialist), if the television is on the blink we have it repaired (specialist), if the body starts to judder we go to a doctor (specialist), and if the mind begins to reel we seek out psychiatry (a specialist). In all of this we act as consumers without an informed view or point of access to what is under the bonnet or inside the box.

It will be argued that it is difficult to keep relating back and forth from the general to the particular. We must have the details apparently since observation of the detail will provide the scientific facts for life. Each time we find a new detail in some sub-sub-sub category of a science we cannot hope to relate it to every other detailed fact and piece of information. And if some new idea emerged from another specialist how difficult it would be if that conflicted with the idea structure that we have built in our own specialised world of study. Often we don't want to look at changes in life for fear that they may demand that we change too.

It has been suggested rather optimistically that western science is nearing the end of the assembly of information. As if the world were really a pile of material to be dug out and sifted through in order for understanding to be achieved! But there is no end to the number of thought forms and there is no end to the possibilities of life. This being so because life is change and change provides new possibilities and potential for life. Only when we stop looking at the details and look at what supplies the details will we understand what we are seeing. Only by perceiving the life force that fills the thought forms will we perceive the process of life.

Essentially this process begs that we work with a different approach. It is the mind that works with this assembly of facts, the ordered argument. But as we know, the argument too quickly runs into debate and discussion; we cannot hold the centre of our thinking. The mind totters without the ordered hierarchy of knowledge.

We must learn to think with our hearts...... The mind says that the heart cannot think......the heart laughs......the mind says that sounds like madness......the heart is open to receive.

The heart knows that all life is one.

8 · *The Need for a New Medicine*

All of this would not be necessary if the other way was working. Quite clearly it is not. This great diversity of ideas and thought forms, the complexity of detail and the rival claims of different viewpoints leave us bemused. But worse than that it leaves us adrift without map or compass. In the days when science could justify itself by demonstrating its successes we had the illusion of purpose but the fact is that things are going wrong, badly wrong. A catalogue of this year's disasters will look mild set against the tragedy of what comes next. It is not going to get better in that way. The signs are writ so large how can we avoid reading them?

What we need is a new medicine. Not a wonder drug, not a surgical implant nor a form of synthetic ego support. We need something that will help us wake up to see what is going on, so that we may see life for what it is. We need to regain our sense of discrimination so that we may once again recognise what is harmful to life and what is of benefit to life. We need something that will help us to understand what we are so that we may simply live. We need something that is not dependent upon the specialist and fragmenting forces of intellectualism, something that works with life as we know it. Something is needed that will help us work with change for it is our inability to go with change that drives us away from life. We need something that will work with the life force within us to bring us to a healthy and happy living. Something that will work in harmony with nature and bring healing to the planet.

9 · *The Medical Discoveries of Dr Bach*

In February 1931 Dr Edward Bach had published his book *Heal Thyself*. The title alone was a challenge to the establishment since his invitation is to patients "so that they may assist in their own healing".[3] In an earlier piece of writing he declared his intention to show "how each of us may become our own doctor".[4] His medical discoveries or rather his discoveries about life patterns and the states of being that humans experience at this time do indeed offer just that: the opportunity for each of us to become our own doctor and to heal ourselves.

When we consider the complexity of scientific medicine and the dangers of modern methods of treatment would we not be wiser to leave matters of health to the experts? Well yes, if we are thinking of using only such methods we would do well to leave them to those who are trained to use them. But there are other ways to health. Dr Bach was quite clear on this. Speaking to a group of homoeopaths at Southport in 1931 he begins:

> ... *I come to you as a medical man: yet the medicine of which one would speak is so far removed from the orthodox views of today, that there will be little in this paper which savours of the consulting room, nursing home or hospital ward as we know them at present.*[5]

or again in his book *Free Thyself*:

> *Health is listening solely to the commands of our souls; in being trustful as little children; in rejecting intellect (that knowledge of good and evil); with its reasonings, its 'fors' and*

> 'againsts', its anticipatory fears: ignoring convention, the
> trivial ideas and commands of other people, so that we can
> pass through life untouched, unharmed, free to serve our
> fellow-men.[6]

And further on in the same chapter:

> Truth has no need to be analysed, argued about, or wrapped
> up in many words. It is realised in a flash, it is part of you. It is
> only about the unessential complicated things of life that we
> need so much convincing, and that have led to the develop-
> ment of the intellect. The things that count are simple, they
> are the ones that make you say, "why, that is true, I seem to
> have known that always," and so is the realisation of the
> happiness that comes to us when we are in harmony with our
> spiritual self, and the closer the union the more intense the
> joy.[7]

Bach did not dwell upon the issue of his disagreement with
contemporary medicine but we know for sure that his ideas had
led him far away from the authoritarian outlook of science and
the authority of specialists. Rather he wanted each of us to take
responsibility for our life and for our health and happiness.

It would be some time before people understood what he
was trying to convey, that he knew. So he spoke to the future:

> The prognosis of disease will no longer depend on physical
> signs and symptoms, but on the ability of the patient to correct
> his fault and harmonise himself with his Spiritual Life.[8]

And speaking of the future for medicine he said:

> The patient of tomorrow must understand that he, and he
> alone, can bring himself relief from suffering, though he may
> obtain advice and help from an elder brother who will assist
> him in his effort.[9]

Lest we think that only medically trained people can be such an "elder brother" he points out:

> *We are all healers, and with love and sympathy in our*
> *natures we are also able to help anyone who really desires*
> *health. Seek for the outstanding mental conflict in the*
> *patient, give him the remedy that will assist him to over-*
> *come that particular fault, and all the encouragement and*
> *hope you can, then the healing virtue within him will of*
> *itself do all the rest.*[10]

By this mention of mental conflict we come upon the essential message of Dr Bach's work – that it is mental conflict that causes illness. We might equally say it is the emotional state or the mental state: it doesn't help to bicker over words for the essential truth of this is to be perceived by the heart and not by the intellect. We can also see from this last quotation that Bach recognised an inherent "healing virtue" that could act within each of us: what we have termed the life force.

All of this, however, shows what came towards the end of Bach's life when he had fashioned the ideas upon which he was to base his new medicine. It is interesting to see how he came to this position where he declared that we must forget the intellectual approach, break free from orthodox ways of working and return to the simplicity of little children. For that we must look back over his life and observe the influences that shaped his ideas.

As a boy Edward Bach was apparently careful and imaginative while being very determined and strong in character. He took great care of his younger sister and was altogether very caring for the weak and those in need. He no doubt saw medicine as a caring profession and determined to become a doctor. He also had a great love for the natural world and the countryside, he was fond of long solitary walks and had a passion for fresh air (he even removed his bedroom window so that it might not become shut!). Strange then that at 16 he left school and went to work in his father's factory: a brass foundry in Birmingham.

For 3 years he was employed in the family business (1903-1906). We may suppose that he learned much. An engineering firm works with strong elemental forces; forging, casting and machining metal has its own poetry and truth. In the furnace of our hearts we forge the cast of our character. A brass foundry is no bad place to see passion fire the cold metal of inherited forms so that they may be melted down and cast into a new shape. Bach witnessed materials changing state, an experience that he was unlikely to forget. But while this and the many other subtle influences of working with people may have formed his character we can see how Bach needed to break free from the assumptions that family karma had put upon him.

It was three years before Edward had finished with his father's business. Ostensibly he worked in the factory because he felt a request for money to train as a doctor would be difficult. Whether we call this pattern false modesty, pride, fear, lack of confidence or indecision is of no consequence – he clearly needed time to grow to be his own man. Family obligations hold many people in the shell of inappropriate behaviour throughout their life. That this issue was important to Bach we can have no doubt for he continually refers to the need to give other people the freedom to choose their course in life:

> *We must earnestly learn to develop individuality according to the dictates of our own Soul, to fear no man and to see that no one interferes with, or dissuades us from, the development of our evolution....*[11]

> *Think of the armies of men and women who have been prevented from doing perhaps some great and useful work for*

humanity because their personality had been captured by some one individual from whom they had not the courage to win freedom; the children who in their early days know and desire their ordained calling, and yet from difficulties of circumstance, dissuasion by others and weakness of purpose glide into some other branch of life, where they are neither happy nor able to develop their evolution as they might otherwise have done.... [12]

Thus the child should have no restrictions, no obligations and no parental hindrances, knowing that parenthood had previously been bestowed on his father and mother and that it may be his duty to perform the same office for another.

   Parents should be particularly on guard against any desire to mould the young personality according to their own ideas or wishes, and should refrain from any undue control or demand for favours in return for their natural duty and divine privilege of being the means of helping a soul to contact the world. Any desire for control, or wish to shape the young life for personal motives, is a terrible form of greed and should never be countenanced, for if in the young father or mother it takes root it will in later years lead them to be veritable vampires.... [13]

The gaining of freedom, the winning of our individuality and independence, will in most cases call for much courage and faith. [14]

He could not tell us more plainly: he is speaking out of personal experience. If it was the idea of the expense that held him back from training as a doctor we can easily understand the problem. He was the eldest son, however, and one suspects that was closer to the heart of the difficulty. But Bach was not a man to be held in the thrall of an idea, especially an idea that was preventing him from achieving what he wanted to do. He made his way to medical school and after many years of study (in 1912) he was 'qualified' – well, he was M.R.C.S., L.R.C.P., M.B., B.S., and D.P.H. It had taken eight years. He was constantly under pressure of work as he had insufficient financial support and was obliged to earn his living as well as work and study. It cost a lot to qualify – it nearly cost him his life.

In 1913 Dr Bach was appointed Casualty House Surgeon at the National Temperance Hospital. He was 27 years old. As a boy his health had been a matter for concern and now he had to give up his post after only a few months owing to illness. As house surgeon he would have been on call day and night working under great pressure where life was often at stake in the casualty department. It may have been exciting but it was also certainly exhausting and nerve-wracking. He could not sustain it. Nora Weeks, who perhaps knew Bach better than anyone, comments in her biography[15] that he had little use for accepted theories which he had not tested and proved for himself. Bach had seen how surgery worked and knew first hand what it was capable of and also its limitations. To many he was in the top rank of his profession where reputation and fame were found but he could not continue. Perhaps surgery did not come easily to him and he was later to eschew even the use of hyperdermic needles in the treatment of illness. However it may have been, this was a turning point in the outward progress of Bach's career in medicine.

When he recovered from his "breakdown in health" he set up in practice in Harley Street. Having gone along the path of working in an institutional set-up (hospital) he tried the same medical principles when applied from his own consulting room. It was not much better. He still found orthodox medicine failed to give sufficient lasting benefit to his patients. Bach was not a person to sit back and wait for answers: when one avenue was explored and found to be a blind lead he started upon the next. Looking at contemporary medical research he thought he might find better results and a more sympathetic methodology in the Immunity School. In bacteriological research many interesting discoveries had been made since the pioneering work of Pasteur and Koch. It was a form of research that was demanding in terms of time and experimentation. But it was in the forefront of medicine and offered new possibilities to Bach.

He took up a post as Assistant Bacteriologist at University College Hospital, London. While he continued in practice he began research. Basically he searched the body tissues and blood of people both healthy and sick to find what bacteria characterised their condition. At its most basic bacteriology searches for the physical organism that causes illness (germ theory). Bach was later to declare that such findings were merely results of illness not the cause. But at this stage it was a more subtle and delicate form of medicine than the use of surgery and was the next step upon his path of realisation.

This was a time of great intensity in Bach's life. At the outset of the World War he had tried to enlist but was considered unfit for service. Bach was disappointed. As for us we might afford a smile for had he been stronger physically he could well have died in Flanders. Instead he tended the wounded in the hospital and was in charge of over 400 "war beds". He also took on more work in the medical school as Demonstrator and Clinical Assistant. He worked and worked. In his researches he came upon a form of intestinal bacteria that were found to be more plentiful in the gut of the chronically ill. He was to prepare a vaccine from these and begin a new form of treatment for such things as arthritis and rheumatism. The results were encouraging.

Yet in all this he cannot have been happy. "We can judge our health by our happiness, and by our happiness we can know that we are obeying the dictates of our souls", [16] he was to write later. Whatever else was happening in his life at this time he was personally in crisis. In July 1917 he began to bleed and fell unconscious. He had cancer.

Many speculations might now be made. But we do not know many of the facts of what was taking place at this time. What of Bach's family, his love-life, his mental state? We do not know what pressures he was working under. War was ravaging Europe and he had been very anxious to fight. Was he finding that his assumptions were being beaten about by reality? It is more likely that this illness was rooted in his personal life. Bach's ideas were forged in the reality of his own experience and later he wrote that:

> *Disease is the result of wrong thinking and wrong doing, and ceases when the act and thought are put in order. When the lesson of pain and suffering and distress is learnt, there is no further purpose in its presence, and it automatically disappears.*[17]

Bach was told that he had no more than 3 months to live. He was given surgery and no hope. What actually happened next we do not know. Again there is the temptation to speculate. He went back to his work with renewed vigour we are told, and as he toiled at it he found that the deadline was passed. But he was working like this before and he had developed the cancer. So work alone would not explain his recovery. Something fundamental must have changed for him during this time. Some new beginning. Some shell of constriction, some mental state that had enslaved him must have given way so that he was able to revivify his body and walk out from the shadow of death. There was some kind of healing.

It is significant that Bach should have met with this difficulty – he now knew from personal experience what it was to be terminally ill and what it was to regain health. He could now speak with the authority of reality, with the knowledge of one who has been there. He was no mere theorist. So he could write:

In true healing there is no thought whatever of the disease:
it is the mental state, the mental difficulty alone, to be
considered: it is where we are going wrong in the Divine
Plan that matters.[18]

The sense of Divine Plan must have begun to figure strongly
for Bach at about this time. He was a Freemason and
strongly committed to the masonic philosophy and inner
teachings. What may his teachers have shown him at this
time? Was this the moment when he struck out for freedom
that he had previously failed to find? We cannot tell. But
again we find in his later writings he speaks quite
emphatically on such matters:

Disease of the body, as we know it, is a result, an end
product, a final stage of something much deeper. Disease
originates above the physical plane, nearer to the mental. It
is entirely the result of a conflict between our spiritual and
mortal selves. So long as these two are in harmony, we are
in perfect health: but when there is discord, there follows
what we know as disease.

Disease is solely and purely corrective: it is neither
vindictive nor cruel: but it is the means adopted by our own
Souls to point out to us our faults: to prevent our making
greater errors to hinder us from doing more harm and to
bring us back to that path of Truth and Light from which
we should never have strayed.

Disease is, in reality, for our good, and is beneficent,
though we should avoid it if we had but the correct
understanding, combined with the desire to do right.[19]

If we dwell upon this issue it is not in order to question
Bach's greatness as a man or the genius of his medical
discoveries. It is rather to illustrate how exactly he knew
what he was talking about. It is too easy for one who has

never had such troubles to tell others how to be free of them. But the realities of common human experience are always recognisable.

At this time too Bach's problems were not merely concerned with his research work and his own health. His first wife, Gwendoline, whom he had married early in 1913, died from diphtheria in April 1917. He remarried in the following month and his illness appeared in July though we may suppose that it had been developing for some time. It is not really very important that we know exactly what was happening at this time. Bach's married life was and can remain a personal matter. What is important is to recognise the emotional pressure that he was experiencing and that he was not merely a medical bystander witnessing the life difficulties of other people.

Bach continued his work as he was convalescing from the operation but in fact he was parting company with conventional bacteriological research. In the spring of 1919 he joined the staff of the London Homoeopathic Hospital. He became involved with a yet more subtle approach to medicine and through his reading of the work of Hahnemann began to see new prospects for reaching to a level of treatment that might truly relate to the causes of disease not merely deal with the effects. He was looking for something we may be sure but it was not going to be found in conventional science:

> The science of the last two thousand years has regarded disease as a material factor which can be eliminated by material means: such, of course, is entirely wrong.[20]

At this time one suspects that Bach's reading and thinking widened to take in things other than medical research. He had a strong interest in the traditions of the east and like many others in the years between the wars he learned from ancient thought a

new way to approach the problems of his day. This is certainly
evident in the ideas that he puts forward though he is discreet in
referring to our western religious teachings and the example of
Christianity. His own words, however, evidence his real
interest:

> *But the times are changing, and the indications are many*
> *that this civilisation has begun to pass from the age of pure*
> *materialism to a desire for the realities and truths of the*
> *universe. The general and rapidly increasing interest exhi-*
> *bited to-day for knowledge of superphysical truths, the*
> *growing number of those who are desiring information on*
> *existence before and after this life, the founding of methods*
> *to conquer disease by faith and spiritual means, the quest*
> *after the ancient teachings and wisdom of the East – all*
> *these are signs that people of the present time have glimpsed*
> *the reality of things.*[21]

It is often noticed that Bach's thinking is very modern and
we may feel that those words have an expression that is more
contemporary to our time than his. Bach was working for
the future. It might be argued that the ways of technology
carried the future, then and now, but ultimately we will
come to see that truth is simple and that there is simplicity in
truth. At a certain level everything is complex and the more
we see the more complex it becomes. But beyond all the
complexity there are the simple truths of the heart, the
simple truths of life. It was these simple truths that Bach was
seeking.

Ten years of research and application in bacteriology and
homoeopathy ended one day when he closed his laboratory,
his clinic and his consulting rooms and left London for good.
It was a drastic change and left his friends and colleagues
amazed. He had made such advances in his work apparently,
he was a famous and respected man, he had money, status

and reputation. All the things that people set in conventional life patterns would wish for. And he threw them all over. What kind of reason might he give for the decision?

> *Be captains of your Souls, be masters of your fate (which means let your selves be ruled and guided entirely, without let or hindrance from person or circumstance, by the Divinity within you, ever living in accordance with the laws of, and answerable only to the God Who gave you your life.*[22]

It is strong stuff. We might ask – did he live by it himself? The answer must be "yes". Bach was a man of vision, guided by a vision and everything he encountered was measured against it in a search for what would answer his need. If he chose to call that 'living according to the guidance of the Divinity within you' he is just trying to keep it simple. He is using the word imagery of his time and the traditions that he knew and loved. We may choose our own.

The guidance that he received in his work had led him to try many different things. He had progressed through conventional medicine from surgery, to bacteriology, he had worked in homoeopathy and looked at many of the novelties of his day like X-rays and even Abram's Black Box. He had researched into diet and its effect upon cancer treatment. But in every case he turned to look forward to new possibilities. Guidance does not necessarily mean that we are taken by the hand and led directly to the realisation. Rather we search through the opportunities that life offers and find always a deeper understanding that will lead to realisation.

For some people homoeopathy is the realisation of the search, the end of the road. It is said that could we but understand it homoeopathy has a remedy for everything – every problem has its pattern; we have only to recognise it, potentise it (prepare it by homoeopathic principles) to the right degree and as "like cures like" all will be well. Bach studied homoeopathy and used homoeopathic techniques in the preparation of some of his early medicines but he was to search further. Why? His writings answer us clearly:

> *It is obviously fundamentally wrong to say that "like cures like". Hahnemann had a conception of the truth right enough, but expressed it incompletely. Like may strengthen like, like may repel like, but in the true healing sense like cannot cure like....*
>
> *Do not think for one moment that one is detracting from Hahnemann's work, on the contrary, he pointed out the great fundamental laws, the basis...we are merely advancing his work, and carrying it to the next natural stage.*[23]

Bach greatly admired Hahnemann's work and followed his intimation that we should look to the personality of the patient rather than the disease. At first, too, Bach followed with the principles of potentising from the material of the substance that characterised the illness: he followed Hahnemann in that he reversed the action of the damaging bacteria by giving them back to the patient in potentised form. But he was to come to see this as fundamentally inappropriate. After all, at what point does the poison become a healing agent? If it is a matter of reversing the action then it would be better to start with the substance that was already the true antidote to the problem. Bach explains the matter like this:

> *And if we follow on this line of thought, the first great realisation which comes upon us is the truth that it is disease itself which is "like curing like": because disease is the result of wrong activity.... it is the very disease itself which hinders and prevents our carrying our wrong action too far and at the same time, is a lesson to teach us to correct our ways, and harmonise our lives with the dictates of our Soul....*

> *Another glorious view then opens out before us, and here we see that true healing can be obtained, not by wrong repelling wrong, but by right replacing wrong: good replacing evil: light replacing darkness.*
>
> *Here we come to the understanding that we no longer fight disease with disease: no longer oppose illness with the products of illness: no longer attempt to drive out maladies with such substances that can cause them: but, on the contrary, to bring down the opposing virtue which will eliminate the fault....*
>
> *True, hate may be conquered by greater hate, but it can only be cured by love: cruelty may be prevented by a greater cruelty, but only eliminated when the qualities of sympathy and pity have developed: one fear may be lost and forgotten in the presence of a greater fear, but the real cure of all fear is perfect courage.*[24]

Taking his instruction from the natural world Bach saw that homoeopathic action was not the way of nature. Darkness is replaced by the light of the sun not by any form of darkness; dryness is refreshed by rain not by any form of drought.

Although homoeopathy has its greatness Bach was guided to the possibility of healing more directly. For this he was to search in nature for the plant forms that held a clear pattern that is the positive antidote to the negative pattern. He had drawn inspiration from the homoeopathic school and his later work was not running counter to homoeopathy. As he put it he wanted only to walk a little further along the road, as indeed we may now be called upon to do.

So Bach left London and began a new life one might say. He had completed his theoretical research and from now onwards in his remaining years of life he was to put into practice the ideas that he had formulated. The shift that took place at this time is more than the assembly of dates. But dates help to put it into perspective:

1928   Shift from potentising bacteria to the discovery of first herbal equivalents.

   Search for suitable plants.

   Realisation that psychological types existed and that they influenced illness.

   Finding Mimulus, Impatiens and Clematis in September.

   Outlines his thoughts to British Homoeopathic Society in November.

1929   Continues in practice but uses new remedies.

1930   Leaves London in May for Bettws-y-coed, Wales.

   Discovery of the "sun method" of potentising.

   Goes to Cromer in Norfolk.

   Writing *Heal Thyself* and other material published in *Homoeopathic World*.

   Finding of next six remedies.

   Putting the Bach Flower Remedies to work.

1931   Travels through England and Wales searching for plants.

1932   Writes *Free Thyself* – an account of the first 12 remedies, later to become *The Twelve Healers & Other Remedies* (1933).

In his search for this new medicine Bach gave up everything he had worked for as a medical doctor. He returned to the instinct of his childhood and roamed the countryside. As a boy of 10 or 12 he had spent whole days walking alone; now a man in his forties he returned to his source. We say he searched for and found the remedies by intuition, often without a realisation of what that means. Bach was clear on the matter: "what is called intuition is nothing more or less than being natural and following your own desire absolutely". For him it was like being a happy child left to live without interference and not interfering, free to be simply alive. Intuition functions automatically when we are in a balanced and harmonious state within ourselves and in relation to our surroundings.

Bach was not entirely alone during this time, however. He had the friendship of several understanding colleagues: among them Nora Weeks and Victor Bullen. To them he confided his ideas, to them he showed the plants and countryside that he loved and to them, eventually, he entrusted the future of his work. Nora Weeks' biography of Dr Bach speaks with an eloquent simplicity of the understanding that they shared though she says nothing of her part in the work. But these friends meant a great deal to Bach in a way that neither of his two marriages had (his second marriage had ended after a few years in agreed separation).

It is to Nora Weeks that we look for an account of how Bach lived and worked during those last years of his life. Bach himself destroyed most of his writings and research notes so we have few documents to testify to his method of working or the way that he found the remedies. This is unfortunate since we are left with a system of medicine finished, complete and satisfactorily proved but somewhat 'up in the air'. It is as if a researcher into genealogy found a couple of generations of the family left without known parents: the children exist but where is the blood line? At a certain point Bach's research took a leap and we find it difficult to see where and how. In 1928 he is walking on one bank of the river still working as a bacteriologist but searching for herbal equivalents to his vaccines and then a leap or rather a series of leaps and he appears on the other bank with a "thin glass bowl" potentising certain flowers that are to hold a new healing power.

Well, we have a choice. We may decide to leave him on his side and say his was an insight and inspiration that is beyond us or we may choose to build a bridge that will take us across to a deeper understanding of how it works and how it is. Those who prefer the first course of action are left with his system of healing and can rejoice in the fruits of his work. An explanation such as it is will be that he was an extraordinarily sensitive man who had wandered and who was led, who found through suffering and personal affliction: a blind and painful discovery. But Bach's work, his writings and his flower remedies invite another view and while it is more demanding it is also more rewarding.

10 · *A Bridge to Life*

"It is impossible to put truth into words",[25] says Bach and
perhaps that is why he whittled his writings down to the
minimum. People who have a familiarity with them will
know of their simplicity. Yet they are still fraught with
structured ideas of Soul and Divinity. Bach sought for words
to describe the simple truth he had perceived in his being
while ultimately the only witness we can have to the truth is
to be there in it ourselves. For that we must stay in being
without thought or judgement seeing life simply for what it
is.

Of course it is not easy. We want answers, we want
structures. If this bridge is to be built it must have founda-
tions of reason and purpose, the building blocks of meaning
and the clear span of intellect. Oh? But they bring tension,
worry, anxiety and uncertainty. Such fixed forms create
stricture and control. Already I begin to doubt my existence,
to doubt my being. It is like...it is like a tight-rope walker
balancing high but beginning to falter when he looks down,
it is fear and doubt that assail him as his foot slips. Such are
the difficulties of the mind.

We should walk, as Bach did, into the fields and then
look again. There we may see that life IS. Do you see the
shift, from inside the head and out into the free spaces of
being? In the field the grass waits patiently in service shel-
tering the earth and its inhabitants; thistles blow their seed,
trees endure the spaces while the crows rattle noisily above
the heads of the sheep. All are just being. We may be
struggling to understand in the noise of our thoughts until

we stop and look outward. Then we may receive the gentle perception of being. Truly the half of our problem is that we try too hard. For understanding is just Being:

> *Consider the lilies, how they grow; they neither toil nor spin; yet I tell you, even Solomon in all his glory was not arrayed like one of these.*

God gave Solomon "wisdom and understanding beyond measure and largeness of mind like the sand on the seashore" and he "spoke of trees, from the cedar that is in Lebanon to the hyssop that grows out of the wall...." He spoke of the natural world and his words were wise. But there is greater wisdom yet in nature itself. There we may perceive our being, not merely hear of it reflected in proverbs and fine teachings. Knowledge is available to everyone of us through the perception of our being. To know what this is we must do it, not think about it. And when we know this we will see the simplicity of it all.

It is the mind that always returns to theories. The heart works in practice. There is a gentleness like soft rain in this truth. And if we doubt its relevance to Bach's work consider: why else did he spend so much time out in the countryside walking, watching, observing and being? He had travelled as far as he might in the realms of theoretical medicine and he then went to contact the only one great healer in this life.

Of course he still had questions. We still have questions. But we know where they must be addressed. That, as we suggested earlier, is the riddle of nature. They will be answered by intuition: which is nothing more than "being natural".

If we wish to cross this bridge and so to cross the gulf of the unknown we need two buttresses to support our plank. They are clear enough. One is self-knowledge, the other a knowledge of nature. One comes with the other, they are not to be seen separately. To put it more simply we need to know what is life. Understand that and we will see well enough how

Bach saw it. Bach tells us this in so many words when he speaks of the education that will be needed by the physician of the future. And let us remember that he said that we are all healers, all able to help ourselves and others – so the education of the physician is the education that we all need:

> *The education of the physician will be a deep study of human nature; a great realisation of the pure and perfect: and understanding of the Divine state of man....*
> *He will also have to study Nature and Nature's Laws: be conversant with Her healing Powers....*[26]

The study of human nature is no great matter, we can study ourselves. And we have ample textbooks in the material that Bach gave us. A study of the 38 mental states that Bach describes in *The Twelve Healers & Other Remedies* will provide us with a complete picture of the dispositions of our nature. That is why he drew up the list! He observed the variety of psychological states and found that they derived from these 38 conditions of "outlook upon life". These negative traits like anxiety, frustration or guilt determine the way that we look from inside of ourselves at the outside world. If we can see and understand the viewpoint or disposition from which we look out upon life we will understand why it is that we have a distorted perception of what life is. Could we but harmonise and balance the outlook through self-realization and self-knowledge we would not see outwardly anything but the simple truth of what life is. Knowing that, we would know ourselves to be one with it – in the unity of life. No more conflict, no more difficulty. Simply being.

The other way around is equally appropriate: we may either feel discomforted with the outer world or with the inner. If we look at nature and see it for what it is, recognising the profound truth and simplicity that is written in every part of the natural world then we would reflect back into ourselves that truth and could not fail to be happy. What we see outside is a reflection of what we are. What we are is a reflection of what we perceive life to be.

> To see a World in a grain of Sand
> And a Heaven in a Wild Flower,
> Hold Infinity in the palm of your hand
> And Eternity in an hour.

Bach puts it a little differently from Blake. For Bach the idea is put into a word rather than an image but the message is identical:

> The development of Love brings us to the realisation of Unity, of the truth that one and all of us are the One Great Creation.
> The cause of all our troubles is self and separateness, and this vanishes as soon as Love and the knowledge of the great Unity becomes part of our natures. The Universe is God rendered objective; at its birth it is God reborn; at its close it is God more highly evolved. So with man; his body is himself externalised, an objective manifestation of his internal nature; he is the expression of himself, the materialisation of the qualities of his consciousness.[27]

If we could develop this love (heart rather than head) and realise this sense of unity (simply being) we would come to recognise how it is. We would become one with life and understand the nature of life and that we are one with it because it is one with us. Then whatever we looked at (outside) we would recognise as part of ourselves (inside). AND THEN we would understand that whatever we experience inside has its equivalent outside. We are no longer stuck with the problem of me and my life because it is all ours and part of the unity.

Returning to Dr Bach and bridge building it may be clear now that he discovered his flower remedies because he allowed the nature of the plant to be one with his nature. He also allowed his nature to find its true equivalent in the plant. Once we stop putting up barriers and shells of separation it is most likely that like will go to like and that we will find what we are looking for. Much of this is so simple that it hardly needs to be said. Why, we know that certain people like certain colours and are naturally attracted to them. Others are drawn to a place they feel related to, or to eat food that will help them. Children know it: they even play the game *What's your favourite colour, what's your favourite flower...?*

If we could retain the simplicity of children we would know instinctively what would make us happy. We still do know it as adults and may think of it as unconscious preference or an intuititive prompting although it is no more than our selves saying "that is what I really want". But we have grown away from our simplicity and our intuitive faculty of "being natural and following our own desire absolutely". We have forgotten the simple joy of living and the happiness that comes from the heart. Rather do we stand on one bank of the river looking with envy and dissatisfaction at this world. Or, looking across the water we gaze with longing to a place where the sun shines but we feel unable to go. The river runs in our land, both banks are of this world but, yes, we need a bridge.

11 · *Healing Herbs*

We are told that there was an occasion in 1928 when Dr Bach had first insight into the way that his work might develop. He had long felt that underlying an illness was the mental outlook of the patient but until this time he had not recognised that the mental state might be classified and formally described. Then one night this famous dinner... was it, one wonders, a masonic occasion? As Nora Weeks describes[28] it we know it changed the course of Bach's work. His thought for the seven bacterial nosodes which characterised seven personality types was reformed so that the grouping would be made not according to the physical landmarks (bacteria types) but the emotional and mental states. A new landscape was to open before him where the manner, mood and mentality of the person were to be seen as the points of reference, not the illness or products of illness.

It was several years before Bach was to declare that he had completed his surveying in this new land . He began at once, however, to put his new ideas to work (never one to hang about) and it was later that same year that he found the first three of the 38 plants that are now so strongly associated with his name. He continued to work with the bacterial medicines meanwhile: his scientific training restrained any impetuosity.

Imagine now his state of mind. He has seen something but as yet does not know what it really is. He knew that he had to follow where it led but this was quite outside the realms of previous research. It was as if he had seen a sketch of a new land but had now actually to draw the maps and plot the landscape. Once more he is starting out afresh and as before he is searching for a more refined system of medicine. Now, however, the laboratory bench must go. No more test-tubes and germ culture dishes. From now on the experiment and the experimenter are one and the same. He became the technician and he became the lab. He has before him the conviction that a new healing agent can be found in the trees and plants of nature and that it must be for the psychological state of human experience not the physical. For the first he went to walk in the fields and for the second he took himself.

The first remedies Bach found were actually seen as equivalents to his bacterial types. He prepared them as he had his vaccines. Later they stayed in his repertory although they were prepared differently. The plants were Mimulus and Impatiens. These would now be seen as descriptive of two differing states: fear of known things and irritability. If the thought is correct that Bach discovered these healing herbs by relating them to the state of his own psyche then we should expect these two flowers to speak of his type. Do they? We can only guess now. But Bach certainly spoke of his own impatience and it is supposed that he was an Impatiens type. And the Mimulus? Perhaps he is not so likely as a candidate for fear, at least not when we read the description as it came to be in *The Twelve Healers*. But this description was refined and altered over a period and if we look at the earlier description in *Free Thyself* then we get clues:

> *Are you one of those who are afraid; afraid of people or of circumstances: who go bravely on and yet your life is robbed of joy through fear;* **fear of those things that never happen; fear of people who really have no power over you; fear of to-morrow and what it may bring; fear of being ill or of losing friends; fear of convention;** *fear of a hundred things?*
>
> **Do you wish to make a stand for your freedom, and yet have not the courage to break away from**

your bonds; if so Mimulus, found growing on the sides of the crystal streams, will set you free to love your life, and teach you to have the tenderest sympathy for others.

This description from 1932 reveals just the negative state of mind that might have held him back from his purpose. If he was thinking of leaving London and giving up his old work what would people think of him, how will he survive, what if he gets ill again and the cancer returns, what will happen to the well-respected Dr Bach? We know now that all would be well but he may have been anxious at the time. Mimulus would have helped him, no doubt. No true researcher would not first test his medicine upon himself and doubtless Bach took the Mimulus. It gave him a quiet courage, control and emotional stability so that he directed his purpose to the future work that he was to do. How beautiful – the first remedy he finds is the one that will give him freedom and help him to find the rest. And the Impatiens? Bach was coming to self-knowledge.

Still the question might be there: how did he find these plants and know that they were the ones to use? If he had watched others at this dinner and seen that they had characteristic types he must have turned the question upon himself. He was watching closely at this time in order to find and evaluate the psychological types. He must have considered his own behaviour as part of that. Then, knowing that he was looking for a flower that was equivalent to that state he had simply to look. First he allowed himself to be drawn by intuition (go where you will), then by attraction he would have seen what he sought.

This process is in fact a commonplace experience in other contexts. We do it with food by selecting from the market or menu, with clothes when we spot a garment that is just right or with gifts when we match the person to the present. Quite simply we carry an image of what we seek (we bear it in mind, have a picture of what we want) and go on matching it against what is available. When we see something we think, yes, that's quite like it or that's it exactly. We match image to object.

For Bach the matching game started with the search for a flower that would bring a gentle, forgiving feeling to the sense of tension and impatience. To understand properly why this plant has such a feeling we need to look at the flower, just as he did. If we do so the true observations that we make of its image and quality are not really described in words. Bach was looking at the subtle form rather than the physical plant. Nevertheless we can observe certain things. Its growth is prolific and fast, it tends to colonise a particular area, amidst the dark foliage the flowers hang as small bursts of colour, delicate and mobile and in seed the pods explode to scatter their contents; all of which has a relationship to the remedy type.

The poet Blake describes the beginning of the more subtle perception when he declares that a plant was outwardly a thistle but "inwardly 'twas an old man grey" (curiously Bach at one time was to think of Sow Thistle as one of the remedies but later abandoned it). Many such ideas are part of our popular folklore. Willows are gnarled and twisted, vengeful and not to be trusted and, as boys should know, are not safe to be climbed. Quite different the Oak, renowned for its stalwart strength, its dependability, the English emblem. Yet while they are strong the oak trees can rot from within and one day fall unexpectedly. Again with Gorse we know that when it's in flower it's kissing time – it's always in flower, it's always kissing time! Just so with hope it is eternal and ever present. A plant like Wild Rose has had a long association with man and in those sad places where tumbled walls mark an old dwelling place wild roses are often found marking the spot where human efforts have turned to resignation.

The physical sight of the plant, however, is different to the metaphysical insight. To understand the nature of a particular flower we must spend time with it, allow its quality to spread into us and fill our being. By merging the inner and outer, realising the unity of things and opening ourselves to the flower we will know it. If, for instance, we stand with our back to an oak tree and allow it to speak to us it tells clearly of its being. It says: "I endure". Through wind and storm, through time and season, with patient purpose and constancy this tree endures. That is its thought.

Going into the place where we may realise that, however, is not always helpful. So a word of warning. If we try this we may find that it is not altogether a healthy experience. In such situations it is possible to lose contact with ourselves, lose contact with the body and our ordinary experience of reality. There is little doubt but that Bach found this to be so. How do we know? Because the third remedy that he found was Clematis which helps those who 'go off' in this way. It helped him to remain earthed and in conscious reality at a time when his mind must have been rather considerably disassociated. Going out into the unity of life is a fine thing but we must be quite sure that we have got ourselves properly prepared for such a journey.

It is not chance then that led Bach to find these first three flower remedies in 1928. Rather they were the ones that he needed to find, for himself. At this date he prepared them in a way that was less potent than his later techniques but the healing force of the plant was still present and still of the same kind. When Bach had found these three remedies he used them in his London practice. During 1929 he tested them on patients and found that they worked effectively. It is interesting to note that these remedies required no experimental testing on guinea pigs since they were in no way toxic. Towards the end of the year he decided to give up using the bacterial vaccines. He now concentrated his efforts on developing his new system of medicine.

Two processes appear to work concurrently for Bach at this time. In one case he is examining and observing the quality of different plants, in the other he is developing his observation of the human states that will become the 'pictures' for the new remedies. We know that he began by looking for twelve remedies for twelve different states and these were to become the original Twelve Healers as they are listed in *Free Thyself*. In this booklet he lists the twelve great qualities that are characteristic of perfection as we see it in the 'Great Masters'. He suggests that these have each a negative condition, the antipathy of the condition that we need to find for the fulfilment of our life purpose on earth. In life we find that the negative state may lead to illness because we are failing to learn the essential lesson of our existence: thus he reasons that it is negative emotional and mental states that cause disease.

These original remedies were all kept when Bach extended the repertory in later years although the key words were slightly modified. The table that he gives in *Free Thyself* [29] has a strong sense of order in it. Here is the feeling of a theory that is going to be amplified. It is like a map with broad delineations: mountains in the north, river and forest in the south: a picture map without the details of contours.

Failing			Herb			Virtue
Restraint	...	...	*Chicory*	...	...	*Love*
Fear	...	...	*Mimulus*	...	...	*Peace*
Restlessness		...	*Agrimony*	...	...	*Peace*
Indecision	...	...	*Scleranthus*		...	*Steadfastness*
Indifference		...	*Clematis*	...	...	*Gentleness*
Weakness	...	...	*Centaury*	...	...	*Strength*
Doubt	...	...	*Gentian*	...	...	*Understanding*
Over-enthusiasm		...	*Vervain*	...	...	*Tolerance*
Ignorance	...	...	*Cerato*	...	...	*Wisdom*
Impatience	...	...	*Impatiens*	...	...	*Forgiveness*
Terror	...	...	*Rock Rose*	...	...	*Courage*
Grief	...	...	*Water Violet*	...		*Joy*

No doubt Bach liked the harmony of numbers and 12 has a great many associations that reinforce it. Although the first twelve have a sort of cardinal quality to them, they are the primary states, the most characteristic types, they do not really cover the full range of human experience.

Bach saw these first twelve as sort of archetypal qualities – Virtues as he calls them. We all need to develop the positive attribute of each of them in ourselves through life on earth, "possibly concentrating upon one or two at a time". For this reason they are sometimes seen as being the type remedies* by which it is meant the twelve essential types of human experience. Somehow this idea corresponds with the neatness of his earlier researches. He maps out a theory and then finds the material to fit it. Although Bach put wonderful and heroic life effort into finding these twelve there is the feeling that the work was relatively pedestrian at this stage when it is compared to the last three years of his life when he was swept away by a force like a tornado of discovery.

A word that is often associated with Bach's research and his discovery of the remedies is suffering. This has come about because his finding of the later remedies, the *Seven Helpers* and then the second nineteen, was attended by a deterioration of his physical health. He used his body as a laboratory and it was damaged by the experience. But it is not helpful to explain his discoveries as the result of suffering. An alternative view would be like this. Bach developed the schema that would show him the first twelve remedies. He recognised in himself the nature of each of these personality types, worked with it, amplified it perhaps and then sought the appropriate flower. Later he came to see that something would be needed for people who had grown beyond the simple 'type remedy' and who were

* The idea has been pointed out by Nickie Murray of the Bach Centre that these are primary states that will be found more readily before our personality is overlaid by difficulty. Because we play games and confuse our simple outlook in life with complexity it is sometimes necessary to look for more subtle states, but the primary 12 remain as the essential types of psychological outlook. The later remedies then appear to derive from these essentials. We are likely to find them more apparent in children, animals or plants.

controlled and imprisoned in a state of mind that had no prospect for release. But of these states he had as yet no personal knowledge; he was not bound up in them himself. He began easily enough with Gorse, Oak, Heather and Rockwater. In each case he was able to develop the picture of what he sought and search for the balancing force. Rockwater we know is not a plant but water that comes from a healing spring. But as the search progressed through 1934-35 he seems to have been swept into states of mind that formed no part of his theoretical scheme. He did not know the nature of the various emotional states that were to be found still less the antidote. With great intensity he would experience the feeling of say mental anguish or depression and then be driven to search for the Sweet Chestnut and Mustard flowers to counteract it.

In all he found 19 new remedies in 1935, experiencing each mood intensely for two or three days before finding the remedy. He had little respite. He did suffer physically at this time but his discoveries were made because of his realisation, not because of the suffering. As a person he was not attached to the process that his body experienced knowing that the reality of life lay not with the negative but with the positive state.

Bach made the observation[30] that a man who was a leader should know more about his subject than his followers and that if one was to be a leader in the struggle against human suffering it would be necessary to have an expert knowledge of the subject. It is true that Bach suffered much pain in his life both physically and mentally but the pain was learning, not a virtue in itself. It is also true that he was a lonely man, especially in the last years of his life. So few people understood his vision or could appreciate what he was attempting to do. Most of his erstwhile friends and colleagues thought he had lost his way. His sensitivity one might say then led him to an Agrimony condition; at the end he appeared to be a lonely eccentric, kindly but seeking for oblivion. His early death may have been a signal that his work was complete but it was also sought as a release from the tension of being that he experienced.

It is important that we remember this now, fifty years on. In the two generations that have passed since his time we have all grown to recognise his greatness and come to understand something of what he was working for. If we now look around there are so many like-minded friends who will share their hearts with us. So many who appreciate the music of the inner world and can offer an open heart to a sister of brother. If we would heal the pain that Bach may have felt we should help each other now.

1928	Sept.	Impatiens		
		Mimulus		
		Clematis		
1930	Aug.	Agrimony		
		Chicory		
		Vervain		
		Centaury	} 12 Healers	First 19 all
		Cerato		potentised
	Sept.	Scleranthus		by the Sun
1931	June	Water Violet		Method
	Sept.	Gentian		
1932		Rock Rose		
1933	April	Gorse		
	May	Oak		
	Sept.	Heather		
1934		Rockwater	} 7 Helpers	
		Wild Oat		
		Olive		
		Vine		
1935	March	Cherry Plum		
		Elm		
		Aspen		
		Beech		
		Chestnut Bud		
		Hornbeam		
		Larch		Second 19 all
		Walnut		prepared by
	through	Star of Bethlehem		Boiling
		Holly		except for
		Crab Apple		White
		Willow		Chestnut
		Red Chestnut		
	to	White Chestnut		
		Pine		
		Mustard		
		Honeysuckle		
		Sweet Chestnut		
	Aug.	Wild Rose		

12 · *Making Bach Flower Remedies*

The order in which Bach found the remedies is of interest. The first twelve formed a distinct group and then seven more were added, then the second nineteen. *(See opposite)*. The preparation of these remedies was of two kinds; by what Bach called *The Sun Method* and *The Boiling Method*. The first nineteen remedies with the addition of White Chestnut (found in 1935) were all prepared by the sun method. The last group of remedies, eighteen of them, were all 'boilers'. There has been a little confusion over this matter of how remedies are prepared. Nothing will make the matter clearer than quoting Bach's own description as published originally in *The Twelve Healers & Other Remedies*.[31] Bach wanted this information to be generally known as indeed he wanted all his writing to be widely available.

METHODS OF PREPARATION
Two methods are used to prepare the remedies.

SUNSHINE METHOD
A thin glass bowl is taken and almost filled with the purest water obtainable, if possible from a spring nearby.

The blooms of the plant are picked and immediately floated on the surface of the water, so as to cover it, and then left in the bright sunshine for three or four hours, or less time if the blooms begin to show signs of fading. The blossoms are then carefully lifted out and the water poured into bottles so as to half fill them. The bottles are then filled up with brandy to preserve the remedy. These bottles are stock, and are not used direct for giving doses. A few drops are taken from these to another bottle, from which the patient is treated, so that the stocks contain a large supply. The supplies from the chemists should be used in the same way.

The following remedies were prepared as above:

Agrimony, Centaury, Cerato, Chicory, Clematis, Gentian, Gorse, Heather, Impatiens, Mimulus, Oak, Olive, Rock Rose, Rock Water, Scleranthus, Wild Oat, Vervain, Vine, Water Violet, White Chestnut Blossom.

Rock Water. It has long been known that certain wells and spring waters have had the power to heal some people, and such wells or springs have become renowned for this property. Any well or any spring which has been known to have had healing power and which is still left free in its natural state, unhampered by the shrines of man, may be used.

THE BOILING METHOD

The remaining remedies were prepared by boiling as follows:

The specimens, as about to be described, were boiled for half an hour in clean pure water.

The fluid strained off, poured into bottles until half filled, and then, when cold, brandy added as before to fill up and preserve.

Chestnut Bud. For this remedy the buds are gathered from the White Chestnut tree, just before bursting into leaf.

In others the blossoms should be used, together with small pieces of stem or stalk, and, when present, young fresh leaves.

All the remedies given can be found growing naturally in the British Isles, except Vine, Olive, Cerato, although some are true natives of other countries along middle and southern Europe to northern India and Tibet.

There follows a list of English and botanical names as is generally known.

Nora Weeks and Victor Bullen shared the ideals that Dr Bach had embodied in his work. One such might be characterised by his phrase "to gain freedom, give freedom" (*Free Thyself* Ch:X). For that reason they published the illustrated guide on how to prepare the Bach Flower Remedies.* It is not possible to quote directly from this book but the directions given there elaborate and clarify Dr Bach's notes. For the present purpose the following observations can be made.

Bach's notes are unclear in respect of the three stages in preparing the remedies: these stages are:

1. Preparing the *Essence*.
2. Dilution of the essence to *Stock* – 2 drops of essence make up into 30mls of stock.
3. Dilution of the stock to *Medicine Strength* – 2 drops of stock make up into 30mls of medicine strength remedy.

When preparing essence it is important to check that the plant is the correct one (more on this below), the flowers should be in perfect bloom and be collected about 9am on a fine bright morning, from as many different plants as possible which are growing in the wild where they have seeded naturally.

By Sun Method

Make the remedy near where the plants grow. No shadow should interrupt the clear sunlight (nor cloud) so the place is important. Fill the thin glass bowl with good spring water and cover the surface with flowers. Avoid touching the flowers by either putting the bowl beneath the plant or covering your hand with a broad leaf and carrying them on that. Leave the bowl in clear sunlight as Bach directs. When removing the flowers use a

---

* In *The Bach Remedy Newsletter*, January 1964, Nora Weeks states explicitly her wish that people should enjoy preparing their own Essences; Vol 3 No.9 p.65.

stem from the same plant and not your fingers! The essence should then be poured into a sterilised bottle that is half filled with brandy. A sterile jug or funnel may be helpful.

By Boiling Method
The same conditions apply to this method. Use a clean saucepan, fill it three quarters full with flowering sprays, leaves and twigs then put the lid on. The boiling is best done at home but make no delay. Cover with two pints of spring water and simmer for thirty minutes. Use a twig from the same plant to press the contents below the water. Afterwards let the contents cool, then remove the twigs and filter the essence. Again half fill the bottle with brandy and half with essence.

These notes are sketchy but the best that can be done at the present time.

Now this essence will make a very large volume of stock. Only a few drops are required to potentise an ounce of brandy in another bottle (stock) and when making up a medicine strength bottle it is diluted again so if we make the essence we have a lot more than is needed individually. That is one thing. Another is this. Some of these plants are now scarce so let us not pillage nature: a flower that is picked cannot become a seed. And thirdly it is important to use the right plant.

Dr Bach tested a great many different plants and concluded that these were the ones that satisfied his intentions. If we find others they too will have a life force that has a notable virtue but it may not be the one that we want or think it is. There can be no doubt that mistakes are easily made. If, for instance, we were to prepare an essence from Bryony thinking it to be Clematis what would be the effect? Bryony is a poisonous creeper that in some ways mimics Clematis but a remedy prepared from the flowers would be rather different and with properties that might not be so pleasant. So care is needed.

13 · *A Definite Healing Power*

The remedies are endowed with a definite healing power quite apart from faith, neither does their action depend upon the one who administers them, just as a sedative sends a patient to sleep whether given by a nurse or a doctor.[32]

Reading what Bach wrote about his work it is interesting to see how he anticipated many of the doubts that might be expressed by other people. That the Bach Flower Remedies might work on what is called the placebo effect is often suggested, at least by those who have not had the experience of using them. But there is no doubt of it, the remedies do have a definite healing power. We must inevitably address ourselves to the question then as to what is this power and how does it work.

Bach's answer to this question is clear enough. He says that the healing power is the gift of the The Creator, it is present in the plant and present in us. He also says that no science or knowledge is necessary in order to gain the benefit of it. Indeed we will gain more benefit from the "God-sent Gift" if we keep it pure, free from science, free from theories: "for everything in Nature is simple". Well enough Bach foresaw the trend of science and the way that technology and scientific research would come to blind us to simple truth.

Yet as we have grown in our knowledge through the expansion of consciousness that has developed in this century so we may better understand what the remedies are and how they work. Bach was concerned that we should not try to use the intellect (science) to understand their action and we could only agree with him. It is not the intellect that will understand their way of working, rather the heart. It has been suggested that by working with the heart we will have a direct perception of what life is through our experience of it. Therefore to think with the heart is to be in the experience (at the heart of the matter) while to think with the intellect is to distance ourselves from the experience and to try to exact a theoretical base from which to make judgements. In any event a 'scientific' approach will not yield much helpful information in this subject. The reason is simply that we have not as yet a science of such subtlety – that is why Bach was led to discover the remedies. They are, in themselves, a science of the metaphysical, the emotional world.

This issue might start to be laboured but it is so fundamental that it is necessary to get it clear. People say that they cannot see how he was able to select and test the flowers that he wanted to use. Why use one form of Gentian and not another? Equally it is asked why there are thirty-eight remedy states rather than any other number. Both these questions can be answered but the answer comes from a view of life that is based upon the truth of the work of Dr Bach. So we might say there are thirty-eight remedy states because there are nineteen manifestations and there are two states for each, one generally internal and the other external. But then we just come to the question of why there are nineteen manifestations!

Earlier it was suggested that all living things are conceived as a thought form that is filled with life force. Plants are no exception. We recognise a plant by its physical form and then by its metaphysical expression (we might recall Shakespeare: "here's Rosemary, that's for remembrance").

When it comes to why Bach chose a particular plant rather than another the answer appears: because that is the plant that exactly represents that thought form. It is true that other plants could be used since they have similar qualities. That is why other researchers, following on from Dr Bach have concluded that certain other plants could have healing essences prepared from them. Of course they can. Every plant has a specific quality, uniquely itself and it is possible to discover its identity and express the thought that it carries. But we must question whether the thought that is held in that form is so universal and succinct that it is really appropriate to all people.

For what Bach did was to describe the universal states of mind that we experience and then find the most exact equivalents of those states in the vegetable world. There are many flowers that may be quite like (Sow Thistle was one) but he wanted to make the match an exact one. It is simple as that: why should we want to make it more complicated by suggesting a lot of inbetween states that are appropriate to a series of flowers that carry a thought form that is not clear?

It seems then that all flowers carry a meaning but in some cases it is clearer than in others and in some cases too it is more specifically appropriate to human patterns of behaviour. When we look at the different forms that occur in trees and plants (vegetable world) we see that some are good for food, some for use in building, some for use in medicine and healing, some for use in less practical and more aesthetic ways (we make music with bamboo pipes). Nothing in nature (or in existence one should say) is without meaning and purpose. We may not as yet know and understand its meaning but since it was conceived as a thought and brought into being and imbued with life we may be sure that it does have meaning. There are other ways of seeing our existence it is true but they begin by denying meaning and therefore can only reduce our perception of what we are. So, as Bach would express it, life is the expression of God, the Creator:

> *All earthly things are but the interpretation of things spiritual.*
> *The smallest most insignificant occurrence has a Divine*
> *purpose to it.*[33]

The simplest explanation of the healing force that is present in these plants then is to say that they carry the purpose of the divine. And indeed they must do: such alone is meaning.

Yet, for reasons that will become clear, it is helpful to describe it a little further. All plants are the result of the thought forms of the planet. They exist where and how they do not by chance but by the concentration of necessary purposes. Let us think why it is that an oak tree, generating many thousands of acorns will not be swamped by its off-spring. It is because that position on the earth for the form of 'tree to be' is currently occupied by that oak: when it goes the next will grow. It is a law of existence that two different beings should not occupy the same space.

We imagine that there is some scientific basis (chemical analysis) that reasons the way plants grow but they have a more subtle meaning in their growth that is in the nature of harmony. It is easy to see that certain plants are dominant (just as certain people are...) but these plants do not overrun the land – why? It is because, if nature is left to herself, the thought form that creates a type of plant colony is in harmony with all the other subtle forces that interplay in that locality. Observation confirms this: we see stands of Pine trees, Mimulus grows in the stony bed of streams, Impatiens with its seeds washed along by the floods lives on the river-banks, Water violet in its secret way hides in the still water courses of fenland.

Some plants will grow in other places as well as their natural habitat. But then the thought form that creates them has not such a strong calling. Heather could be persuaded to the rockery in a town garden but its instinct is for the mountainside. Gentian or Centaury will be found among gravel and tall grasses but the pattern that is true to its nature is on the thin soils and short grass of chalk downs. Sweet Chestnut will grow on chalk and clay but its nature is for sand. It is more than geology that informs these plants and trees. On the mountainside it is bracken that is dominant but yet it does not overrun the heather.

When men interfere with nature the harmony of plant ecology is upset, however. We decide that we will grow what we want where we want it and an altogether different process is created. This is not necessarily wrong or bad it is simply that man creates a thought form that is different to the thought form of nature. If we threw the seed down and accepted the outcome we would find some plants were accepted by the land while others were not. But we tend to work by confrontation and conflict and will it differently.

Where plants grow by nature, however, they partake of the subtle qualities that characterise that exact place. Various names have been used to express the meaning of this. Let us say that the earth carries a pattern of life force that is expressed through the plant as a thought form. If we go to that plant we will have the possibility of contacting that pattern of life force. Just as we are drawn to certain places that are special for us or carry a healing quality that we are attracted to, so the earth carries a force pattern that is attractive for that life form: the plant. If we want to contact that quality we could touch the earth at that place, have a picture of it or somehow take into ourselves the thought form that characterises it. The flower essences work like this.

The life force that is in the plant takes up the pattern that in physical terms we call by a botanical name. But it is more than the physical form just as we are more than the physical body. The thought form that the plant represents has an equivalence to us since all life is one. Nature in its multiplicity and variety is an expression of what man is in a united form (that is the riddle of nature). So the plant carries an exact expression of something that is a general part of mankind. If we need to contact and invoke the pattern that the plant carries we go to the plant.

If we just contact the plant we can feel and share its thought. Bach, however, wanted to get a stronger charge than this and to concentrate the patterned life force ("power") that the plant carried in such a way that we might take it with us wherever we go or take it to those who cannot get out into the fields. The sun method of potentising was to do just this. He saw its significance in the way that it combined the four elements:

> *The earth to nurture the plant, the air from which it feeds, the sun or fire to enable it to impart its power, and water to collect and be enriched with its beneficent magnetic healing.*[34]

As usual we can agree that the method is simplicity itself. What happens is that the life force in the plant is given up into the water so that the water (essence) now contains the thought form, just as the flower did. Is it too much to believe? A reel of celluloid film can carry many thousands of thought forms, a family snapshot holds the pattern of a group of beings, an old shoe carries the memory of dancing, the scent of the past lingers on in life. Such things are part of daily experience.

14 · *The Consolidation of a Mental Attitude*

*Disease is a kind of consolidation of a mental attitude…and
it is only necessary to treat the mood of a patient and the
disease will disappear.*[35]

Using slightly different words Bach repeats this message
time and again. Our mental outlook or emotional state is the
cause of illness. Fear, greed, uncertainty, fixity, guilt, apathy, forcefulness, worry… these are the mental attitudes. As
these patterns of activity become habitual so they constrict
the flow of life force in our bodies and we are prey to illness
and disease. More than that the pattern of mental activity,
because it is causing disharmony in life needs to be corrected
and so it will be brought to our attention (consciousness) for
us to work upon it. Illness is therefore the opportunity for
looking at the truth and encountering change.

In the picture that Bach draws of existence we see that
subtle forces create a pattern, that pattern shapes the material
of life in itself to create a physical result. The process is like
the growth of all life forms. Constant suspicion or jealousy
creates a pattern of behaviour in our daily life, it also sets up a
pattern of activity in our subtle body (the emotional level)
that channels and patterns the life force within us. That
pattern is not a balanced or harmonious pattern. We call it a
negative pattern of behaviour and it deeply influences all our
life. In time it will result in a physical debility or distortion of
health. The negative pattern also acts like a vortex that draws
the material of disease into itself. At a simple level we

recognise this when we think of tiredness as weakening our defences to the common cold. But every other negative pattern of emotional behaviour is also likely to weaken our defences.

The way that negative patterns act upon the body (both physical and emotional) can be visualised. A shock will tear the fabric allowing life force to flow out like blood from a wound. Rigid mental attitudes progressively remove the suppleness from the body just as ageing makes the bones brittle as the structure of the collagen changes (collagen is the elastic fibre in bone and tissue). Fear restricts the flow of life force so that change is less possible just as it creates shallow breathing and so reduces the exchange of gases. The effect of this can be traced through the whole metabolism: less oxygen means less activity in all parts of the body, less red blood (and so the pallor of fear), less efficient digestion, poor circulation and so cold, fatigue and poor health are inevitable. These are all physical effects of a poor pattern of breathing. But the breathing is a result of a more subtle cause – the restriction of the life force that a prolonged pattern of fear or nervousness will induce. It is possible to counteract the effects by learning to breathe better, by taking exercise and so on. This will effectively unsettle the pattern. But if the fear remains the pattern will reform and the condition will continue.

Other problems can be seen in a similar way. A pattern of health often has a quite logical sequence in it if we can ascertain the stages that lead to the originating cause. Any of the feelings of apathy, hopelessness or dejection will lead to a slowing of all life activity in the body, it will be a matter of which form of disease takes hold first when we come to give a name to the illness. Often there are many. In cases where tension, anger, dominance and pride are at work the life force is put under pressure, channelled into a fixed direction. The result is that pressure is localised in the physical body: in the heart maybe, or in the head.

Dr Bach saw this process as being a very literal indication of life activity. It will be necessary, he said, "to be able from the life and history of the patient [person] to understand the conflict which is causing the disease or disharmony...to give the necessary advice and treatment for the relief of the sufferer".[36] For Bach the relationship was direct. If we suffer pain it is because we cause pain to others...it has a slightly judgemental ring to it but he makes his point.

> *Pain is the result of cruelty which causes pain to others, and may be mental or physical: but be sure that if you suffer pain, if you will but search yourselves you will find that some hard action or hard thought is present in your nature: remove this, and your pain will cease. If you suffer from stiffness of joint or limb, you can be equally certain that there is stiffness in your mind; that you are rigidly holding on to some idea, some principle, some convention may be, which you should not have. If you suffer from asthma or difficulty in breathing, you are in some way stifling another personality; or from lack of courage to do right, smothering yourself. If you waste, it is because you are allowing someone to obstruct your own life-force from entering your body. Even the part of the body affected indicates the nature of the fault. The hand, failure or wrong in action: the foot, failure to assist others: the brain, lack of control: the heart, deficiency or excess or wrong doing in the aspect of love: the eye, failure to see aright and comprehend the truth when placed before you. And so, exactly, may be worked out the reason and nature of the infirmity: the lesson required of the patient: and the necessary correction made.[37]*

This idea is elaborated in *Heal Thyself*. It is a little confronting perhaps but Bach wants us to take up the responsibility for our health and for our life. It is our mental attitude that is to be examined not the righteousness of our souls. To him, as both a doctor and as a man, the state of bodily health is a matter of observable fact not something that requires moral criticism. This is important since it is at the heart of the matter. If we judge the body of ourselves or another with the sharp knife of our minds we will only cause pain. We need a loving, caring understanding to appreciate how the mental attitude has become consolidated into this pattern of difficulty. Nothing sentimental will help but a truthful acceptance of life and the will to work with change. If we approach the matter with criticism and judgement we will find it rebounds: we must then examine ourselves to see what is happening.

> *If we have in our nature sufficient love of all things, then we can do no harm; because that love would stay our hand at any action, our mind at any thought which might hurt another. But we have not yet reached that state of perfection; if we had, there would be no need for our existence here. But all of us are seeking and advancing towards that state, and those of us who suffer in mind or body are by this very suffering being led towards that ideal condition....*[38]

It is clear that all of us in life are pretty much in the same boat. It is not a matter where some of us are perfected and others are not. For, as one teacher put it, if we were too good for this world we may be sure that we would be adorning another! So in this matter it is not a judgement that is sought but an understanding of the process of disease.

In order for us to see that what Bach describes is actually so we must observe its truth in our own experience. In such circumstances case histories do not prove anything, rather we must actually see the process for ourselves. For this we must first suspend disbelief and then open our hearts to life: we will be shown. We might perceive by intellectual reasoning but the process is far more difficult. But for those who like to think about it we could go back to the most perfect case history of all, our own life. What we then might see is how the process of our health has reflected the mental attitude that we have had in our lives.

What actually happens then is something rather like this. As we experience life certain patterns of behaviour become engrained in us. They are the responses to a combination of factors: the inherited patterns that dispose our nature to certain attitudes, the learned instinctive responses of family patterning and then the responses that we have to the variety of life experience. What mental attitude these create will be individual for each of us but it will be well established in most of us long before we are adult. Let us suppose that a child finds life to be difficult. Perhaps a deep conflict has developed between the parents. When there is a prospect of the conflict being repeated the child has anxiety. It might displace this mental attitude with pretence, manipulative behaviour, whatever. But in individual cases the physical body could eventually register the story as earache, eczema or enuresis (bed-wetting). In fact each of these three offers a possibility of viewing the way that the pattern is manifesting since bed-wetting is likely to demonstrate fear or anger against the father, eczema a smothered fear and mental turmoil and earache a pressure of anger that wishes not to hear.

If we work with Dr Bach's flower remedies we could prescribe for such a situation and know that as the emotional conflict was eased then the physical problem would disappear. If the mental outlook is no longer being informed by the difficulty then the physical body has no longer that negative pattern distorting the flow of the life force. So while we may begin by attempting to remove the eczema from a suffering child we must actually work to ease the mental outlook. The remedy in such an instance would be Agrimony which is for the anxiety and inner pain that is hidden by the appearance of cheerfulness. In such an example the pain is not allowed to show on the outside emotionally but it cannot be prevented from appearing physically.

In actual fact it is not really necessary even to take a remedy for the difficulty that we experience once we can see that it derives from this mental state. It is quite possible to work directly upon the mental state ourselves once we recognise that it is creating the distortion in our pattern of health. Perhaps we may think that it is asking too much of a child but in fact the child will find it easier to do than an adult because the adult is more bound in with the idea of being unwell. This interestingly is equally true of our responses to actually taking the Bach Remedies for children respond more readily than adults in most cases.

As adults we seem to feel we need something more complicated than this to explain health and illness. We feel that it cannot be so simple. Our instinct is for complex explanations since simple truths are more difficult to avoid. But what Bach is putting forward is a view that requires us to reorientate our ideas. Just as thought forms and karmic shells create the patterns of behaviour that we express in life so we have certain set attitudes about what constitutes health and what leads to illness. These attitudes often require complex intellectual structures to maintain the distance between idea and reality and to distance us from our responsibility for our own life. It is the complexity that leads us to go to specialists.

At the extreme we see all the hardware of the modern hospital system probing, measuring and assembling as many facts as possible in the hope of it making sense. But while modern medicine has successes in some areas it cannot offer any hope of reducing the burden of illness or increasing the prospect of health since it has no explanation as to why we get sick. In other areas of medicine or health care we see that a less technological approach touches more upon the human aspect. But often the problem is still made into a complex issue. The complexity makes it special and enforces the relationship of illness and health that already exists. What we see then is a mental outlook that is structured into the very way that we all see illness: we have a set idea of what our illness is and how we imagine we can get better.

This may be illustrated by the picture that we have formed (mental outlook) about ourselves if we are a patient or a practitioner. Even if we leave out the white coats we have an image where the patient is seen in a recumbent position, lying down under illness. It has to be that way otherwise we have no way of telling who is the patient. It also signifies that the illness has reached a stage of development where we can no longer maintain our daily living in the way we are accustomed, standing on our own two feet. Just the act of seeking help means that we have admitted that illness has got on top of us. For this reason we define a relationship that puts the helper as being okay and ourselves as being in trouble.

The natural consequence of this is to see health as an either/or situation and to imagine that we need only take something to get us up and better again. But while we may receive specific help from another person the process of life is really not built upon such a see-saw. If it helps to think in terms of visual models we can imagine the matter not as a line where we cross into ill health but as a circular image where the centre is the abundance of life and the periphery the various negative states of difficulty. Then, in order to be more in the state of health we need only look to see what leads us towards the centre where there is a greater abundance of life. Any other involvement in the difficulty is just delaying the change.

There are many ways of expressing this. Swami Sri Yukteswar (1855-1936) says:

> *There are two ways to be rid of disease, a right and a wrong way, the one being slow and uncertain and the other being speedy and sure; the foolish physician studies disease*

*in order to bring about health while the wise physician studies
health in order to annhilate disease, saying to his patients:*

*"Fulfill the condition of health and diseases will fall away
from you of their own accord."*

*And if this is so with the body, in like manner is it also
with the mind which is full of maladies in the shape of hatred
and jealousy and sensuality and anger and other painful and
bitter sensations.*

And how will we do this? He says:

*Imagination is the door through which disease as well as
healing enters. Disbelieve in the reality of sickness even when
we are ill; an unrecognised visitor will flee.*

From this we can only conclude that what we each hold in our
minds is the mental outlook that defines our perception of life.
If we hold the attitude that sees ourselves as unable to overcome
our life difficulty then certainly we will be incapable. If we hold
in our mind an attitude that is destructive to life we can only find
ourselves being destroyed.

15 · *You Have Got the Idea*

It is now widely accepted that a good diet is helpful to a healthy life. We are beginning to see the need for such a review of our emotional diet. A meal of artificial feelings, overdone attitudes and cold lifeless caring will not be helpful, especially if we pour on the salt of fixity and the vinegar of suffering. Everything in the physical realm has its equivalent in emotional terms. Even the first-aider's kiss of life has its counterpart in emotional first aid. There is no substance without the thought form that is behind it. Just as we have come to trace the difficulty that is caused by a diet that is imbalanced, heavily saturated by fat, starch and sugar so we will recognise that an emotional outlook that is strongly held by negative thought forms will cause us ill health. An emotional block is a constriction of the life force as surely as a blocked trachea restricts the flow of air or arteriosclerosis and atheroma constrict the flow of blood.

Once we have got this idea one of two things are likely to happen. We may look positively upon the prospect of working so directly upon our health and life. Alternatively we may react emotionally to the idea. If we start to look at it this way we might well feel that we are to blame for the mess, we might feel guilty for our failures and begin to reproach ourselves for what we feel we have done to our life and to others. Understandable response. But it is itself a negative emotion and we can actually be free from it. The lessons of life are not intended to induce guilt, rather to help us to be happy. So we need to begin by lovingly accepting ourselves and not feeling guilty for what has happened. Life has mystery in it still and nothing is made clear and no problem solved by dealing out blame.

It is inevitable that in life we make mistakes and it even appears to be that we must make mistakes and will go on being given life difficulty until we see and admit that we do. The issue is then not one of blame for making mistakes but what we do when we find out our failings. The ideal might be that we stay balanced in a loving acceptance of life but usually we topple over into a pattern of negative emotion. Each of us has a tendency to topple a particular way. That tendency shows our disposition to the remedy types that Dr Bach delineated: the 38 remedy states.

We might see it like this. As people interact with life there are inevitable tensions and difficulties that arise. They are part of the dynamic of life experience. In some cases we turn away from the life force as it enters into us since it can be painful, in others we accept the life force but cannot utilise it effectively. As we 'rub off' our difficulties upon one another so negativity can arise between us emotionally like static electricity. The pattern of fear or hopelessness, the pattern of irritation or indifference, indeed any of the human states of mind, builds as a voltage charge in our being. As the static builds we find it increasingly difficult to hold the charge.

Sooner or later the static must be earthed out. We use the force of this static charge to create thought forms. These thought forms could be positive or negative in content but since they arise from the friction or pain of contact they tend to be negative. We then look for an opportunity to unburden ourselves of them. We can do this to one another or agree to do it to the third party (scape-goating). If we wish to we can project them over a considerable distance to another person though the effect of 'earthing' is lessened and slower then.

If we witness the earthing out of these thought forms we will see the life force dissipate in the drama of the exchange. If we are disposed to irritation there will be an outburst – sparks will fly. If we are disposed to self-pity we will collapse in floods of tears. If we are fearful we will find the difficulty builds until we get to the point where what we feared actually occurs (we have created the reality from the charge). Alternatively we may bury it in our guts where it festers as resentment, or we may attempt to smother it and suppress the force until it explodes. If apathy is the response then we allow the charge straight through us so that the life force ebbs away – even those who come near to us will be earthed out by the pattern so that they will leave depleted.

Quite often we get drawn into life dramas that will force us to work with these difficulties. In terms of the remedies we often recognise that in relationships people actually work the pattern together. Thus a Vine person who is domineering requires a Centaury person to order about. The Centaury person who is weak-willed equally needs the bossy Vine for the expression of the life lesson. In the same way the Chicory type needs someone to be Chicory with: the emotional binding must be made upon someone. So life provides an external expression for the thought form – hurdles for those lacking in confidence, loads for those who are burdened by life and worries for the anxious. What would we do if we had no problems? We would invent them!

To begin to clear the pattern and all the attendant problems we have only to start work upon it. Changing our diet begins with the first meal. What is required is that we act to change our thought forms and as we change into a more harmonious, positive, life-affirming outlook so we will be well. First we will notice the change as we become happy. Negative thought forms create unhappiness and as they change so we become happy. Then, whatever ill has taken hold of our body it will be eased. Even if the process of degeneration has gone to a point where it is irreversible still the heart will be eased and a gentle and positive acceptance of life will suffuse the body.

A simple and practical way to set to work upon ourselves is through the use of the Bach Flower Remedies. Bach discovered the remedies to help those who were sick in the body but we now can see a way to use them to heal the balance of the mind even before the body becomes an expression of a disease that requires healing. Taking a flower remedy can help us to contact the positive force of life that will counter the negativity. In that case the static charge will be neutralised in us, not earthed out through another person nor turned inwards to cause internal suffering.

It is also possible to work directly with the life force so that we can neutralise the negativity in ourselves, or that which comes towards us. Essentially all that we need for this is a recognition that the negative and positive states exist. Then, instead of building the negative thought form and earthing it out on another person, we can consciously neutralise it by creating the positive thought form. If we are handed the negative thought form of another person the same applies. We can create the positive thought form in ourselves first to neutralise and then to broadcast the force outwards.

In practice what must we do? First let us look again to see what would be the action of the flower remedies. If we are stuck in a pattern that is refusing to work with the forward movement of life experience, where we are constantly look-ing back, rerunning the film of memories with a longing for the happiness of the past then we are refusing to be active in the present. This Honeysuckle state as Bach identified it has a romantic nostalgia. To take Honeysuckle as a Bach Flower Remedy would act to bring us to life in the present, conclude the lessons in the past and to free us from the binding of memories. In consequence the life force coming into us would be used to enhance the present and not feed the thought forms of the past.

In such a case as this the negativity is not an active force that is earthed painfully upon another person but a drawing force that sustains the images of the past. Yet the action is deadly. It works to maintain thought forms that would naturally decay, to keep in life things that should be dissolving back into other levels of existence. It is not so sweet.

If we used Bach Flower Remedies to work on such a state we would find help. But once we recognise that the process is built upon thought forms we would find meaning. We can work directly upon the thought forms themselves. This means that we create thoughts that are the opposite: in the positive of Honeysuckle they are seen as moving into the present and deliberately creating thoughts that are here and now. The example of a different remedy will serve to further illustrate the process. For the Cerato state which in a negative form is imitative and uncertain we can create positive thought forms that will determine that the intuition is responded to, decisions are made and held to. The positive thought form of the tired and weak will be for strength and so on.

However, these thought forms are more than words. They are actual force patterns. It takes an act of will to create such things and it requires our constant effort to sustain them. Bach describes the process:

> *We must steadfastly practise peace, imagining our minds as a lake ever to be kept calm, without waves, or even ripples, to disturb its tranquillity, and gradually develop this state of peace until no event of life, no circumstance, no other personality is able under any condition to ruffle the surface of that lake or raise within us any feelings of irritability, depression or doubt. It will materially help to set apart a short time each day to think quietly of the beauty of peace and the benefits of calmness, and to realise that it is neither by worrying nor hurrying that we accomplish most, but by calm, quiet thought and action become more efficient in all we undertake....and though at first it may seem to be beyond our dreams, it is in reality, with patience and perseverance, within the reach of us all.*[39]

In this way we can bring ourselves to really learn what the Bach Flower Remedies can teach us. For while they are always of benefit as a physical helper the true virtue of the remedies is in their showing of the mental states and how we may each work with them for ourselves. Whether we begin with affirming the positive idea of the state, by contemplating the image of the flower, by attuning ourselves to the natural world, whatever way we endeavour to work we are trying to move towards a harmony of understanding. Bach said that disease was only here in order to help us to see the nature of our conflicts. Equally the substance of any thing is only here to lead us towards the idea so that we can see and understand how it is. If we see and understand already we can do without the substance. If we work with the substance we will come to understand. That is the story of life.

In our world, animals are subject to the limitation of the thought forms that create them. We see animals as bounded by instinct for this reason. A tiger is held within the pattern of its nature just as a gull is patterned to its gull behaviour. The same is true of the animal level in humans. This means that we are bounded by the limitation of our ideas. We can be caught in the web of thought forms such as illness and health, in conflict and violence, in the ideas of polarity, in the concept of materialism that gives us the appearance of being subjected to materiality. But it is actually possible for human beings to realign their being by reference to new or different thought forms. A donkey will always be bound into the limited thought form of donkey: a human being has the potential to transcend.

By consciously creating a new thought form for our being we can change what we are. If our thought form does not contain the illusion of our difficulties they will not exist. In terms of this animal-level problem of illness we can create the thought form of health and realign ourselves accordingly all the way through to the physical. Dr Bach showed us that disease derives from the negative emotional states and that positive emotional states lead to happiness, health and well-being. As such he was aligning himself with a long tradition of wisdom that has always known that mankind creates its own difficulties and has the power to overcome them.

We all know that human individuals are capable of change. As we change as individuals so the world will change. The quality of our thought forms creates the quality of our life. It is our thought forms – yours and mine – that will help to determine what happens. For every thing there is a season, a time when this thing alone is right and proper. Who can stand in the way of an idea whose time has come? It will explode into the public consciousness and no pattern of restraint will withstand it. Life is about change and a love of life brings a joyous exclamation of being without limitation. We must love life more than conflict, we must love life more than illness, we must love life more than unhappiness, we must love life more than any fixed pattern of ideas. Then we may love and accept the life lesson for our being and rejoice in the experience of being alive.

—❦—

NOTES

1 This title is borrowed from a book by Aubrey Gaulter published in 1929 by J. Whitaker & Sons Ltd, London. The subtitle reads "Being the Natural Religion of Truth by Evolution". It is an extraordinary book.
2 *Book of Job* 12:8
3 *Heal Thyself*, Dr Edward Bach; C.W.Daniel Co.; 1931, p.5
4 *Free Thyself*, Dr Edward Bach; 1932, Introduction. [See *Flowers to the Rescue,* Gregory Vlamis; Thorsons Publishing Group, 1986, p.131 *seq.*]
5 *Ye Suffer From Yourselves*, Dr Edward Bach; 1931, p.1[See Vlamis *ibid* p.117 *seq*]
6 *ibid* p.7
7 *ibid* pp.7-8
8 *ibid* p.8
9 *ibid* p.9
10 *Free Thyself: opcit* p.25
11 *Heal Thyself: opcit* p.25
12 *ibid* p.25
13 *ibid* p.26
14 *ibid* p.28-9
15 *Medical Discoveries of Edward Bach, Physician*, Nora Weeks; C.W.Daniel Co.; 1973, p.17
16 *Free Thyself: opcit* p.7
17 *Ye Suffer from Yourselves: opcit* p.3
18 *Free Thyself: opcit* p.24
19 *Ye Suffer from Yourselves: opcit* p.5
20 *ibid*
21 *Heal Thyself: opcit* p.7
22 *Ye Suffer from Yourselves: opcit* p.14
23 *ibid* p.4
24 *ibid* p.2 ff
25 *Free Thyself: opcit*; Introduction

26 *Ye Suffer from Yourselves: opcit* p.8
27 *Heal Thyself: opcit* pp.55–56
28 Nora Weeks, *opcit* p.7
29 *Free Thyself: opcit* p.19
30 *See* Nora Weeks *opcit* pp.138–9
31 *Twelve Healers & Other Remedies*, Dr Edward Bach;
     C.W.Daniel Co.; 1936
32 *Free Thyself: opcit* p.19
33 *ibid* p.5
34 *The Homoeopathic World* 1930; "Some Fundamental
     Considerations of Disease & Cure"; Dr Edward Bach.
35 Dr Edward Bach quoted by Nora Weeks:
     Medical Discoveries of Edward Bach, Physician; opcit p.57
36 *Ye Suffer from Yourselves: opcit* p.8
37 *ibid* p.6
38 *Heal Thyself: opcit* Ch:III, pp.14–18
39 *ibid* p.51